5-
Back
Relief

Karen Sullivan

Royal College of
General Practitioners

HarperCollins Publishers Ltd
77–85 Fulham Palace Road
London
W6 8JB
www.collins.co.uk

First published in 2007
Text and illustrations © 2007 HarperCollins Publishers

10 09 08 07
7 6 5 4 3 2 1

ISBN 978-0-00-725159-9

Designed by Martin Brown
Thanks to Dr Rodger Charlton FRCGP
Printed and bound in Italy by Amadeus

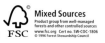

Mixed Sources
Product group from well-managed
forests and other controlled sources
www.fsc.org Cert no. SW-COC-1806
© 1996 Forest Stewardship Council

The information (including without limitation advice and recommendations) contained in this book is presented for general information purposes only. It is in no way intended as advice for any individual problem or to replace the professional medical care and/or services from a qualified health care practitioner. The information in this book cannot and should not be used as a basis for diagnosis or choice of treatment. Always seek the advice of your doctor or other qualified health care provider with any questions you may have regarding a medical condition and prior to starting any new treatment.

Collins uses papers that are natural, renewable and recyclable products made from wood grown in sustainable forests. The manufacturing processes conform to the environmental regulations of the country of origin.

CONTENTS

INTRODUCTION	4
BACK BASICS	6
EVERY DAY BACK RELIEF	38
MEDICAL HELP FOR BACK RELIEF	81
BACK RELIEF THROUGH EXERCISE	94
ALTERNATIVE METHODS	140
FURTHER RESOURCES	186
INDEX	190

INTRODUCTION

Back pain, especially pain in the lower back, is one of the most common health problems in adults around the world. Fortunately most back pain is temporary, resulting from short-term stress on the muscles or ligaments that support the spine, rather than from a serious injury or medical condition such as nerve damage or kidney disease. But whatever the cause, and however short term the symptoms may be, the pain can be debilitating and, in the UK, results in over 11 million days off work every year and some 7 million visits to the doctor. Employers lose up to £335 million every year, and the cost to the health and community care services is over £1 billion.

According to the most recent statistics supplied by the UK Health and Safety Executive, back pain affects as many as four out of five of us. Other research shows that almost half of the adult population in the UK reports lower back pain lasting for at least 24 hours at some time during the year. In almost 80 per cent of cases, the problems recur, impacting on the lives of millions of sufferers.

The good news is that there is plenty that you can do to prevent back pain from becoming a chronic problem, to ease the symptoms and to make a successful recovery – all by investing just a little time every day. Even those of you who have never been affected by back pain, but wish to improve the health of your back to prevent future problems, will benefit from the information and advice in this pocket-sized book.

Some of the exercises and programmes in this book may take a little time to learn – and you may need a little help from a practitioner or expert to get you started – but once you've mastered the basics, you can expect to make real progress in only five minutes a day.

Some of the advice and exercises will work as a short-term fix for acute pain; others will improve your back pain over time while making a big difference to your mobility, well-being, energy levels and the way you feel every day. There are a wealth of treatment options and restorative programmes in this book – and you can pick and choose between them, according to your individual needs. Take time, too, to learn the secrets of a healthy back and how to prevent back pain from recurring in future.

Whether this is your first port of call before visiting your doctor, or you plan to use it alongside treatment, it's never too early to get started. And with this book, you'll be on the road to recovery – in just five minutes a day.

BACK BASICS

Understanding how your back works and what can go wrong can make a big difference to the way you treat and use your back, and to how you view your symptoms. A little knowledge gives you the power to make changes that will – in many cases – relieve pain instantly, and in others help you to make progress towards a pain-free life.

The back is a complicated structure and many things can go wrong; some are more serious than others, and we will look at those here. However, even minor injuries or problems can cause excruciating pain in sufferers; it pays to know what to expect and how to get the appropriate treatment, whether you choose conventional or more alternative methods.

We'll look at how to get your back problem diagnosed, and what to expect from the variety of different treatments now available. Most importantly, perhaps, we'll look at prevention, because taking steps to keep your back strong and healthy can not only prevent short-term back pain, but also ensure that problems do not recur in the future.

THE HEALTHY BACK

The back is an intricate structure of bones, ligaments, muscles, nerves and tendons. The backbone, or spine, is made up of 33 bony segments called *vertebrae* (*see* figure on p. 9). The vertebrae are arranged in a long vertical column and held together by ligaments, and are attached to muscles by tendons. Between each vertebra lies a gel-like cushion called an intervertebral disc, consisting of semifluid matter surrounded by a capsule of elastic fibres. Between the vertebrae are joints, called 'facet joints'.

The discs absorb shock from the changing weight loads applied to the spine from excessive – as well as normal – activities such as walking, running, lifting and so on. The spine's four natural curves also help to distribute these loads evenly, while providing structural support and stability. Facet joints and the discs allow the spine to bend and twist. Different muscles coordinate movement in many directions.

The spinal cord is an extension of the brain that runs through a long, hollow canal in the column of vertebrae. The meninges (the three membranes that cover the brain and spinal cord), cerebrospinal fluid (the fluid that bathes the brain and spinal cord), fat and a network of veins and arteries surround, nourish and protect the spinal cord.

Thirty-one pairs of nerve roots emerge from the spinal cord through spaces in each vertebra. These form the 'peripheral nervous system', or PNS, which is effectively the part of the nervous system outside the brain and spinal cord. The central nervous system (CNS) is comprised of the brain and spinal cord itself.

The PNS conveys sensory information from the body to the brain and instructions for the body to move, from the brain. In a healthy back, the nerves emerge easily and are not 'trapped' or restricted by muscles, the vertebrae or the discs, and therefore do their job without any pain or discomfort. A healthy back is both flexible – to provide movement and motion – and stable – to provide balance.

A healthy back is a balanced back: your cervical (neck), thoracic (chest) and lumbar (lower back) curves are all properly aligned. (You know your back is aligned properly when your ears, shoulders and hips are 'stacked' in a straight line.) A healthy back is also protected and supported by its flexible, elastic discs and well-conditioned muscles.

Once you understand how your back works, and what can go wrong, you're ready to start taking care of your self. By using proper posture (when you sit, stand, lift, recline and move) and by exercising the muscles that support your back, you can prevent the most common causes of backaches. The result is freedom from back pain and a stronger, healthier back.

WHAT GOES WRONG

As we age, our spines change and the normal 'degenerative processes' can affect the vertebrae, facet joints and discs. Trauma (such as injury), wear and tear, disease, lack of exercise and poor body mechanics (posture, lifting, bending, etc.) can alter the structural integrity of the spine, causing pain, discomfort and damage.

Pain is a symptom rather than an illness, so the important thing that you and your doctor will need to work out is what is causing the pain, and also what caused the problem in the first place. Pain can be 'referred' from other sites in the body, including organs. For example, appendicitis, kidney disorders, pelvic or bladder infections, period pains, ovarian disorders and even aneurysms can cause pain to be referred to the back.

The parts of a healthy back

cervical spine

thoracic spine (area of upper back pain)

lumber spine

coccygeal vertebrae

Common causes

Most back pain is not serious and usually resolves within a few weeks – without treatment. Common 'non-specific back pain' can develop in association with a number of causes, including muscle strain, minor injury to the back, overuse, muscle disorders, pressure on a nerve root and poor posture. Pregnant women, smokers (*see* p. 33), construction workers and people who do repetitive lifting all have increased risk of back pain.

When to see your doctor

If you are a regular back-pain sufferer, you may well be used to the symptoms, and have painkillers or a series of exercises or techniques to relieve the discomfort. This book is a good choice for you because, not only are there a variety of methods to deal with back pain, but also many ways to improve the health of your back. Unfortunately, as most of us learn, age does cause degeneration, and things 'give', rupture and strain more easily; in fact, studies show that over the age of 30, things take a turn for the worst and back pain is just one result of the normal degenerative process. So, while some back pain can be expected, and while there are many things you can do to combat this on your own, there are also times when you must see your doctor.

These include where:

- The pain persists for more than a few days.
- One of your 'regular' bouts of back pain doesn't resolve within a few weeks.
- Painkillers, stretching and gentle exercise don't help.
- The pain wakes you at night.
- You have difficulty controlling your bladder or bowels.
- You have fever, chills, sweats or other signs of infection.
- The pain feels different to other back pain.
- You notice other unusual symptoms.

Strains and sprains

The most common cause of back pain (in some 50 per cent of cases) is an injury to a muscle (strain) or ligament (sprain). Strains and sprains can occur for many reasons, including improper lifting, excess body weight and poor posture. They can also develop from regularly sitting awkwardly, carrying something heavy, sleeping at an odd angle or, of course, as a result of an obvious injury. Because it is a pivot point for turning at the waist, the lower back is particularly vulnerable to muscle strains. In some cases, pain is felt immediately upon lifting or turning; sometimes pain follows later on. Injured muscles may also stiffen or 'knot', which is effectively a self-protective mechanism that prevents further damage occuring to your back.

SERIOUS BACK CONDITIONS

Prolapsed disc

Over time, normal wear and tear can cause one of the discs between the vertebrae in your spine to rupture (herniate or 'slip'). Prolapsed discs are found in about 30 per cent of adults above the age of 20, but only about 3 per cent of sufferers produce classic symptoms (such as sciatica; see opposite). Due to degeneration of the disc, you may have done nothing outside your usual activities to cause it to go. However, exceptional strain or injury to the area – or the back in general – can also cause a disc to rupture. Back pain results when the herniated disk pinches one of the nerves that come out of the spinal cord.

disc

A prolapsed or herniated intervertebral disc can put pressure on the nerves that branch from the spinal cord, causing pain, numbness and tingling. It can also cause swelling and muscle tension in the area.

nerve

spinal cord

disc

Discogenic back pain

Discogenic back pain is thought to be a common cause of lower back pain. Discogenic back pain is the result of damage to the intervertebral disc, but without disc rupturing. Diagnosis of discogenic back pain may require the use of a discogram (*see* p. 19).

Sciatica

The sciatic nerve, which runs from your spinal cord to your leg, is most likely to be affected by a ruptured (slipped) disc. Compression or inflammation of this nerve causes sciatica – a sharp, shooting pain in the lower back, buttocks and leg.

Sciatica is known as a 'nerve root syndrome', which produces different kinds of symptoms to muscular or tendon problems. There can be numbness along the course of the nerve's pathway. Nerve root syndromes occur when the nerve is 'impinged' (touched) by, say, a rupture or bulging of a disc, or compression of the vertebrae. This syndrome can also be caused when there is muscular injury to the area, which causes swelling and inflammation that effectively 'traps' a nerve.

Spinal stenosis

Spinal stenosis is a narrowing of the lumbar (back) or cervical (neck) spinal canal, which causes compression of the nerve roots. Spinal stenosis mainly affects middle-aged or elderly people. It may be caused by osteoarthritis or Paget's disease (which affects bone growth, see p. 16) or by an injury that causes pressure on the nerve roots or the spinal cord.

Rheumatoid arthritis

Arthritis most commonly affects joints such as the knees and fingers; however it can extend to any or all joints in the body, including the small joints (facet joints) in the back, causing pain and inflammation and affecting movement.

Osteoarthritis

Osteoarthritis of the spine is a degenerative condition that causes slow deterioration of the discs. Without the cushioning that these discs normally provide, the joints between vertebrae press tightly against each other. This can cause back pain and stiffness. The body may try to compensate for these changes by building new bone (spurs) to support the area where loading pressure is increased. Osteoarthritis usually develops over many years of physical activity; obesity and injury to a joint are other risk factors.

Spondylolisthesis

Spondylolisthesis is a condition in which a bone (vertebra) in the lower part of the spine slips forward and onto a bone below it. In children, spondylolisthesis usually occurs between the fifth bone in the lower back (lumbar vertebra) and the first bone in the sacrum area. It is often due to a birth defect in that area of the spine, which makes it weak.

In adults, the most common cause is degenerative disease (such as arthritis). Other causes of spondylolisthesis include stress fractures (commonly seen in gymnasts, football players and weightlifters) and traumatic fractures. Spondylolisthesis may occasionally be associated with bone diseases. Symptoms may include lower back pain and pain in the thighs and buttocks, stiffness, muscle tightness and tenderness in the affected area.

Osteoporosis

Osteoporosis is a condition in which calcium is lost from the bones, lowering their density and making them porous and brittle. If you have osteoporosis, daily lifting and other routine activities can cause low back pain by fracturing the front part of the weakened bones. These are known as compression fractures. A fall can have the same effect.

Fibromyalgia

This chronic condition is characterised by fatigue and pain in the muscles, ligaments and tendons – including those of the lower back. Diagnosis of fibromyalgia usually includes a history of at least three months of muscle pain accompanied by pain and tenderness in at least 11 of 18 'tender points' on the body.

Cauda equina

This syndrome is a medical emergency. Disc material expands into the spinal canal, which compresses the nerves. A person would experience pain, possible loss of sensation, and bowel or bladder dysfunction. This could include inability to control urination (causing incontinence) or the inability to begin urination.

Other causes

There are other causes of back pain. Rarely, back pain may indicate a more serious underlying problem such as an infection, diabetes, kidney disease or cancer. Other skeletal causes of low back pain include:

Osteomyelitis (an acute or chronic bone infection, usually caused by bacteria; affected bone may have been predisposed to infection because of recent injury);

Sacroiliitis (an inflammation of one or both of the sacroiliac joints, which connect your lower spine and pelvis; this condition is difficult for doctors to diagnose, and it may be mistaken for other causes of low back pain);

Paget's disease (a disease characterised by excessive breakdown of bone tissue, followed by abnormal bone formation. The new bone is structurally enlarged, but weakened and filled with new blood vessels);

Tumours (possibly cancerous).

DIAGNOSIS

The causes of back pain can be very complex, so it is often very difficult to get an accurate diagnosis for back pain. It is, however, important that you see your doctor to rule out potentially serious illnesses.

Seeing your GP

Your doctor will have a series of questions about how and when your symptoms started, and about the type of pain that you are experiencing (whether it is constant, burning, sharp, aching, etc., and where it takes place in your body). Most doctors will take a thorough medical history, and then undertake a physical examination. This can usually identify any dangerous conditions or family history that may be associated with the pain. They'll ask about pain and other sensations in different parts of your legs, feet and toes. In some cases a 'pinprick' is used on the back of your leg or foot to check that your reactions are normal. Muscle strength may also be tested, and your doctor can ask you to push against his or her hand. Most doctors will test the reflexes in your knees and ankles by gently tapping with a small hammer – just below the kneecaps and above the heels.

Doctors often use the 'straight leg test' to help ascertain whether or not you have a damaged disc.

Your doctor may ask you to lie on your back and then raise the painful leg, without bending your knee. Most people with a damaged disc get sciatica (a pain that runs down one leg) before their leg is two-thirds of the way up, which indicates that a slipped (herniated or ruptured) disc is likely.

In most cases, these types of tests will determine whether or not there is a serious problem and, as discussed earlier, you are likely to be reassured that your back pain is the result of a sprain or strain, poor posture or lifting, muscled spasm or a minor injury. Most back pain will clear up on its own. You may be given some painkillers and some advice on how to look after your back, including some simple exercises (see p. 96).

If, however, your doctor suspects that your back pain may have another cause, or if your pain doesn't resolve within a few weeks, you may be referred to a specialist, who will use a variety of different tests to work out the cause.

Blood and urine tests: these may be offered if your doctor suspects an infection or a condition like arthritis, or after everything else has been ruled out.

X-rays: a conventional x-ray uses low levels of radiation to project a picture on to a piece of film (or electronically onto a computer) and it is used to view the bones and bony structures in the body. It's often used if your doctor suspects that you may have broken bones, injured vertebrae or osteoarthritis. Injured muscles and ligaments or painful conditions such as a slipped disc are not visible on conventional x-rays.

Enhanced x-rays: provide more information than a conventional x-ray, and include:

Discography: which involves injecting a contrast dye into a spinal disc believed to be causing back pain. The dye outlines the damaged areas on x-rays taken following the injection.

Myelograms: contrast dye is injected into the spinal canal, allowing spinal cord and nerve compression caused by slipped discs or fractures to be seen on an x-ray.

Computerised tomography (CT): this quick and painless process is used when disc rupture, spinal stenosis or damage to vertebrae is suspected. X-rays are passed through the body at various angles and are detected by a computerised scanner to produce two- or three-dimensional images of internal structures of the back in 'slices'. It can even reconstruct a three-dimensional model of the spine, which can be rotated and visualised from all directions.

Magnetic resonance imaging (MRI): is used to check for bone degeneration or injury or disease in tissues and nerves, muscles, ligaments, and blood vessels. This test involves placing the patient into the area of a very strong magnet and then measuring the emitted radiation from their body as the magnetic field is turned off. Very precise images of the various structures in the body can be obtained through this technique.

Electrodiagnostic procedures include electromyography (EMG), nerve-conduction studies, and evoked potential (EP) studies:

EMG assesses the electrical activity in a nerve and can detect if muscle weakness results from injury or a problem with the nerves that control the muscles. Very fine needles are inserted in muscles to measure electrical activity transmitted from the brain or spinal cord to a particular area of the body.

Nerve-conduction studies use two sets of electrodes that are placed on the skin over the muscles. The first set gives the patient a mild shock to stimulate the nerve that runs to a particular muscle. The second set of electrodes is used to make a recording of the nerve's electrical signals, and from this information the doctor can determine if there is nerve damage.

EP tests involve two sets of electrodes. One set stimulates a sensory nerve and the other, placed on the scalp, records the speed of nerve-signal transmissions to the brain.

Bone scans are used to diagnose and monitor infection, fracture or disorders in the bone, such as osteoporosis. A small amount of radioactive material is injected into the bloodstream and will collect in the bones, particularly in areas with some abnormality.

Scanner-generated images are sent to a computer to identify specific areas of irregular bone metabolism or abnormal blood flow, as well as to measure levels of joint disease.

Thermography involves the use of infrared sensing devices to measure small temperature changes between the two sides of the body or the temperature of a specific organ. Thermography may be used to detect the presence or absence of nerve root compression.

Ultrasound imaging uses high-frequency sound waves to obtain images inside the body. The sound-wave echoes are recorded and displayed as a real-time visual image. Ultrasound imaging can detect tears in ligaments, muscles, tendons and other soft tissue masses in the back.

TREATMENT

The treatment you receive will depend entirely upon your diagnosis, and all conditions require a slightly different approach. Most back pain can be treated without surgery, and in the majority of cases without any intervention at all. The main aim of most treatment is to ease the pain and any inflammation while the body heals. It is also aimed at restoring proper function and strength to your back, and to prevent recurrence. For many sufferers, however, the pain can be intense and debilitating, whether the problem is serious or not, and self-management can be a frustrating task.

The most important thing you can do in advance of treatment is to avoid lifting, try as hard as you can to maintain regular activities, and take gentle exercise. We'll look at the efficiency and use of some of the more common treatments later on in this book, as well as some tried-and-tested techniques to ease back pain completely.

Medication/drugs

Medication is often used to treat both acute and chronic back pain, and you may be given several options that include both prescription and over-the-counter drugs, perhaps in tandem with external medication. Because many people do end up taking a combination of different things, it is extremely important that you check with your doctor or pharmacist to ensure that you aren't taking too much of any one thing, or that they don't counteract each other's effects. Many drugs are not appropriate during pregnancy or while breastfeeding, or for anyone with liver problems.

Over-the-counter painkillers and anti-inflammatories (non-steroidal anti-inflammatory drugs, or NSAIDs) are taken orally to reduce stiffness, swelling and inflammation, and to ease mild to moderate back pain. Those with asthma or gastro-intestinal problems should use NSAIDS with care. These include ibuprofen, naproxen, aspirin and paracetamol.

Topical analgesics (such as ibuprofen gel or cream) can reduce inflammation and stimulate the blood flow, as well as relieve pain. Others come in the form of a cream or a spray to stimulate the nerve endings in the skin with feelings of warmth or cold, which dulls the sense of pain. These are known as counter-irritants.

Muscle relaxants are sometimes prescribed in the treatment of acute back pain in an attempt to improve mobility and your range of motion (which is often limited by muscle spasms); this is believed to interrupt the 'pain-spasm-pain' cycle – and to make it easier to do some therapeutic exercise.

Anti-convulsants are a type of anti-seizure drug used to treat certain types of nerve pain.

Some doctors prescribe low-dose antidepressants, particularly tricyclic antidepressants, because they have been shown to relieve pain. Antidepressants alter the levels of brain chemicals to elevate mood and to dull pain signals, as well as help with sleep. There is not a convincing amount of evidence that they are of use, but the area is still being studied at present.

Strong painkillers known as opiates (including codeine, for example) are often given in the case of severe, short-term (acute) back pain, or for short periods in chronic back-pain sufferers. Treatment must be supervised by a doctor because of possible addiction, impairment of judgement and other side-effects, such as constipation (which can exacerbate back pain). Some experts believe that these drugs, when overused, can lead to depression and increased pain. Antibiotics could be used if there is an infection of any nature.

Spinal injections

A steroid (corticosteroid) can be injected along with a local anaesthetic into the affected areas of the spine to reduce inflammation and ease pain. For pain relief, injections can be more effective than an oral medication because they deliver medication directly to the part of the back causing the pain. Depending on the type of injection, some forms of back-pain relief may be long lasting and some may be only temporary. There are several types of spinal injections used for pain relief, including epidurals, selective nerve root blocks (SNRBs), facet joint blocks, and sacroiliac joint blocks. Your doctor will be able to explain any of these more fully and suggest the most appropriate treatment for you.

Physical therapy

Exercises and physical therapy are often advised, particularly when back pain recurs frequently or lasts for long periods. In general, the goals of back-pain exercises and physical therapy are to decrease back pain, increase function and provide you with a maintenance programme to prevent further recurrences.

There are many types of physical therapy, including 'passive therapies' (thus called because they are 'done to' the patient), such as heat and ice packs, ultrasound or TENS, and 'active therapies', which are necessary to rehabilitate the spine. Active therapies can include stretching exercises (see p. 107), strengthening exercises (see p. 96) and usually some low-impact aerobic conditioning such as walking, cycling or swimming.

Manipulation

Spine adjustment (manipulation), by an osteopath (*see* p. 146), chiropractor (*see* p. 144), or a physical therapy spine specialist is often recommended, particularly in the case of chronic problems. In some cases, there is a noticeable improvement after just one visit, although more treatment may be required.

Braces

After injury or surgery, moving your lower spine can delay healing of fractures. Braces can be used to limit the motion of the spine, which enhances bone healing, and usually decreases pain and discomfort.

Some braces are rigid; others work more like corsets. People with jobs that involve heavy lifting also sometimes wear corset braces. These braces essentially work by limiting motion and acting as a reminder to use proper body posture when lifting heavy objects.

Alternatives: when back pain does not respond to more conventional approaches, patients may consider other options, such as acupuncture (*see* p. 178), TENS (*see* p. 83) and more. We'll look at some of these in the Alternative Methods section (p. 140).

Surgery

Surgery is rarely needed for lower back pain.
Even if you have a herniated disc or nerve damage,
you are likely to improve without surgery. In serious
cases, where the condition does not respond to
other therapies, surgery may relieve the pain, but
healing can often take months and there may be a
permanent loss of flexibility. There are many types of
surgery, including artificial discs, fusion of the
vertebrae and decompression of the discs. If surgery
is recommended, you'll be advised of the options
and potential side-effects.

PREVENTION

While most back pain does resolve itself eventually, the discomfort, lack of mobility and effect on quality of life can make even short-term problems difficult for sufferers to cope with. And given that the chances of recurrence are high, there is no doubt that prevention plays an important role not only in ensuring that problems don't start in the first place, but also that they do not return. For this reason, doctors provide careful guidelines for protecting your back, alongside any treatment offered.

There are clear ways to prevent back problems, and most of these will also help to ensure that your back stays strong and healthy as you grow older. Later on in the book, we'll look at how to put some of these preventative tips into action in just a few minutes a day.

✔ Warm up before activity. Beginning any activity with 'cold' muscles and joints puts you at risk of injury.

✔ Keep your spine flexible and muscles surrounding it strong by keeping as active as possible. Even if you suffer from regular bouts of pain, exercise – in particular, regular walking – and activity will help. Bed rest is no longer considered an appropriate cure for back pain.

✔ As you become older, if you have suffered from back problems in the past, or if you have had periods of prolonged inactivity, choose regular low-impact exercise, such as swimming, cycling or walking (even speed walking). Just 30 minutes a day can increase muscle strength and flexibility (*see* p. 94).

✔ Consider exercises such as yoga, Pilates or qi gong to help stretch and strengthen the muscles and improve posture (*see* p. 44). This is particularly important as we get older.

✔ Strengthen your abdominal and back muscles. The abdominal muscles support the lower back. People with weak abdominal muscles tend to suffer from back pain and are more susceptible to injury.

✔ Strengthen your leg muscles. The leg muscles play an important role in helping you to maintain good posture and mobility. And strong leg muscles can take much of the burden off your back when you're lifting heavy items.

✔ Reduce stress (*see* p. 39). Stress increases tension in all your muscles including your back.

✔ Avoid slouching when sitting or standing (*see* p. 46). Your back supports weight most easily when curvature is reduced.

✔ At home or work, make sure your work surfaces are at a comfortable height for you (*see* p. 30). This also includes things like your kitchen counters or work bench.

At work

Sit in a chair with good lower-back support and proper position and height for the task. Keep your shoulders back. Switch sitting positions often, and periodically walk around the office or gently stretch muscles to relieve tension. A pillow or rolled-up towel placed behind the small of your back can provide some support. If you must sit for a long period of time, rest your feet on a low stool or a stack of books. The most important adjustments are:

Seat height from the floor – the feet should be able to rest flat on the floor. However, this doesn't mean the feet should always be flat on the floor. Legs should be free to stay in different positions.

Depth from the front of the seat to the backrest – sitters should be able to use the backrest without any pressure behind the knees.

Choose the height of your work surface according to what you'll be doing – the idea is that you should never be crouched over. If you are standing, you will need a higher surface than you would if you were sitting at a desk. Ideally, your work surface should be at the same height as your elbows, whether standing or sitting, and several centimetres below this if it holds a keyboard. If sitting, adjust the seat of your office chair so that the work surface is elbow-high.

A fist should be able to pass easily behind the calf and in front of the seat edge to keep the back of the legs from being pressed too hard and the feet from swelling. Two fingers should slip easily under each thigh. If not, use a couple of telephone books or a footrest to raise the knees level with the hips. Stare straight ahead and relax your body. Where your gaze naturally falls should be the place to put the centre of the computer screen. Raise it using books or a stand if required.

✔ If you sit, you need to move around! In addition to helping the muscles relax and recover, this alternately squeezes and unsqueezes the intervertebral discs, which results in better filtration of fluids into and out of the cores of the discs. Discs stay plumper and, in the long run, healthier.

✔ Wear comfortable, low-heeled shoes. Shoes should be well balanced, flexible and most certainly comfortable. Good shoes provide not only protection for your feet, but also a supportive base that helps the spine and body remain in alignment. Selection of the right shoes, and correctly using inserts if needed to provide even further balance, can help you avoid muscle strain and possible injury.

✔ If you carry a shoulder bag, switch sides often to avoid stressing one side of the back.

✔ Sleep on your side to reduce any curve in your spine. Always sleep on a medium firm surface (*see* pp. 64–6). Using the right mattress and pillow will support the spine so the muscles and ligaments can be stress-free and have a chance to be relaxed and rejuvenated.

Lifting

Always be sure to bend at the hips – not the lower back. Most people believe bending their knees will ensure a safe lift, but this can still lead to a back injury. The most important tip is to bend the hips and push the chest out, pointing forward.

Bending the knees alone will still allow a person to curve the back and risk an injury, but keeping the chest pointing forward will guarantee a straight back. The back muscles will then be used most effectively for maintaining good posture, as they are designed to do. The knees will bend automatically so the muscles of the legs and hips will produce the power for lifting correctly.

Keep the weight close to your body. The further an object is held from your centre of gravity, the more force is required to hold it up.

Do not try to lift objects too heavy for you.

Do not twist when lifting. The shoulders should be kept in line with the hips to avoid this.

✔ Maintain proper nutrition and diet to reduce and prevent excessive weight, especially weight around the waistline that taxes lower back muscles. Weight really does matter! Try carrying a backpack with a 6-kg (14-lb) weight in it, and see how it affects your posture, balance and back muscles. If excess weight is concentrated in the stomach area, even more stress in placed on the lower back.

✔ Make sure your diet has plenty of calcium, phosphorus and vitamin D to help to promote new bone growth – and to ward off osteoporosis. There is also some evidence that antioxidants (*see* pp. 61–2) can help to slow down some of the degenerative effects of ageing, many of which affect the spine.

✔ If you smoke, quit. Smoking reduces blood flow to the lower spine and causes the spinal discs to degenerate. It also increases bone loss, which can lead to osteoporosis. What's more, the action of lighting a cigarette and smoking it can affect posture as you hunch over.

✔ Keep a positive attitude about your job and home life; studies show that people who are unhappy at work or home tend to have more back problems and take longer to recover than people who have a positive attitude.

✔ Listen to your back. Pain is a warning sign. Your

body is telling you that you have already caused, or are about to cause damage. If what you are doing hurts, then stop immediately. There is no truth to the idea that painful muscles are being toned or strengthened. Pain means damage.

✔ Age need not be a barrier to healthy exercise but as we become older our bodies begin the natural process of degeneration, and this includes our spines and the all-important discs between the vertebrae. Slipped discs are more common after the age of 30, so tailor your activities accordingly. While someone may sneeze and rupture a disc when it takes a bungee jump to cause the same damage in someone else, it pays to be careful.

✔ Drink plenty of water. There are several studies showing that dehydration can be a cause of back pain.

✔ Remember that most back pain resolves on its own without intervention, so don't panic. But do see your doctor if your pain is unusual or sends up a red flag (see p. 11).

In the car

The way you sit when you drive can either contribute to or alleviate back pain, and if you travel long distances behind the wheel it's even more important to get your posture right.

It is important to sit with your knees level with your hips. If necessary, use a rolled-up towel or a commercial back support placed between the lower back and the back of the seat for more comfort and support of the natural inward curve of the lower back.

Sit at a comfortable distance from the steering wheel, with your hands in the '2 and 10 o'clock' position and your elbows relaxed. Reaching increases the pressure on the lumbar spine and can stress the neck, shoulders and wrists, and sitting too far away can aggravate back pain. However, it's not a good idea to sit too close either, as you will be more likely to sustain an injury from the car's airbag if there is an accident. Experts recommend that you keep about 25 cm (10 in) between your breastbone and the cover to the airbag for safety reasons.

Before you get out of a car, move your seat back away as far as it will go, and open the door all the way. Place your left hand on the steering wheel and your right hand on the edge of your seat, next to your right thigh, or on the edge of the car roof.

Lift both legs off of the floor, keeping them together, and move your legs and upper body as a single unit towards the open door. You should feel like you are spinning on your bottom; there should be no sensation of 'twisting'.

Next, put your feet on the ground and use your legs, hands and arms to raise yourself out of the car. Push off with your hands from the seat or the door frame, whichever gives you better leverage. Keep your back straight and your head loose and facing forward.

To get back into the car, take these steps in reverse, making sure that you 'spin' rather than 'twist'.

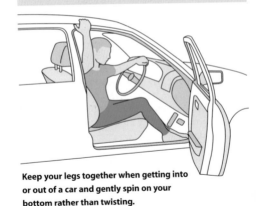

Keep your legs together when getting into or out of a car and gently spin on your bottom rather than twisting.

Travelling

Pack light and use more than one bag. Lifting one heavy bag can be all it takes to cause back pain and problems.

Experts recommend moving slowly when lifting a heavy piece of luggage and breaking the action into smaller parts whenever possible. For example, when lifting a bag into an overhead bin, it can first be lifted to the top of the seat, then into the bin in a separate motion. Similarly, loading a suitcase into the boot of a car can be broken into steps, such as lifting it first to a chair or stepstool, then lifting it into the boot.

Bring your own back support for cars, trains, planes, etc. to support your lower back. Support your feet on a firm surface to prevent stress being transferred to your lower back. Use a footrest if the seat is too high. Your knees should be at right angles to the floor. Choose luggage on wheels and switch hands for pulling it. Stop and turn rather than trying to turn in motion.

Move as much as possible. Sitting in one position for extended periods of time stiffens the back muscles. Get up, stretch and move around every 20 to 30 minutes if possible. Movement stimulates blood flow, and blood brings important nutrients and oxygen to the structures of the back, helping prevent soft tissues in the low back from stiffening and aching after sitting.

EVERY DAY BACK RELIEF

The way you choose to live your life can have a dramatic impact on the health of your back as well as the pain you experience. So not only can you help to prevent back problems, and their recurrence, by adopting a few key measures on a day-to-day basis, you can also help to relieve back pain in just five minutes a day.

Little things like learning to become more resilient to stress, and how to release tension when you do become stressed, adopting a safe position for sex, eating properly to ensure the health of your bones, and even choosing the right mattress and pillows for you can not only make life easier on your back, but help you to deal with the reality of back pain. Small adjustments to your posture and five-minute exercises or once-a-day measures to relieve pain can improve mobility and also prevent future problems. In some cases, you'll find that pain vanishes almost instantly.

And if you are pregnant, this chapter has a few tips to get you through the aches and pains the natural way, and help you to enjoy your new baby without putting more pressure on your back.

DE-STRESS YOUR BACK

Managing stress is important in the treatment and prevention of back pain. Stress can cause and exacerbate back problems for a number of reasons. First of all, when we are under pressure (stressed), stress hormones are released, in particular, adrenaline. One of the things that adrenaline does in the body is to increase our perception of pain. So, in other words, pain that might have been niggling or irritating when we are calm, becomes magnified when we are stressed. These same hormones also cause the muscles to tighten – as we enter 'fight or flight' mode – a throwback from the days when we were stressed for physical reasons, such as being threatened by a wild bear. In some cases the muscles tense to the extent that they go into painful spasm. Back and neck muscles are particularly sensitive to the effects of stress.

When our muscles tense, the flow of blood to the tissues is reduced, which means that they get less oxygen and fewer nutrients. This not only delays healing in the back, but it also prevents acidic waste products from being flushed from the tissues. A build-up of these products can cause fatigue and pain.

In someone with previous back problems, for example, scar tissue from an old injury, or degeneration of the spine and/or discs due to ageing, even the slightest muscle tension can trigger pain and cause further injury or restriction of movement. In fact, the slightest muscle tension may literally be the 'straw that breaks the camel's back', causing a flare-up of sciatica when nerves are compressed, for example, or putting pressure on a disc that was already weakened, causing it to bulge or 'herniate'.

In many cases, stress also creates a cycle of pain and tension that is difficult to ease. Muscles tense because of stress, causing pain; the body reacts to pain by tensing muscles. And, of course, when muscles are tense the back is less flexible and more susceptible to injury through simple things like lifting, or even sitting for too long in one place.

The second important element about stress-related back problems is the idea that emotional and psychological factors are at the root of the pain. The link between emotions and pain have been firmly established through years of research, but the idea that emotional factors, such as stress, are the *prime* influence in back pain is fairly new. In other words, it is believed that some stress-related back pain is in fact psychosomatic – or an illness in which the physical symptoms are believed to be the direct result of psychological or emotional factors. So the emotional aspects of stress either cause or maintain a back problem. This doesn't mean that the pain is all in the mind; far from it, in fact. It simply means that the very real physical symptoms experienced are affected by emotional factors.

This is a complicated and sometimes controversial theory, but with stress and back pain on the increase, one which is becoming increasingly credible. Dr William Deardorff, an American clinical psychologist, explains how emotional health can impact on back pain (see **www.spine-health.com**). He writes:

> In most theories of stress-related back pain, the pain cycle continues and is exacerbated as the pain leads to the patient becoming timid and anxious about daily activities. The pain cycle is characterised by:
>
> The patient becomes unnecessarily limited in many functions of daily life, as well as leisure activities. This decrease in activities is due to the patient's fear of the pain and injury.
>
> This fear may be made worse by admonitions from doctors (and/or family and friends) to 'take it easy' due to some structural diagnosis (which may actually have nothing to do with the back pain).
>
> The limitations in movement and activity lead to physical de-conditioning and muscle weakening, which in turn leads to more back pain.
>
> This cycle results in more pain, more fear, and more physical de-conditioning along with

other reactions such as social isolation, depression and anxiety.

Relieving stress can reduce pain that is aggravated or caused by tense muscles.

Managing stress on an ongoing basis may also help prevent back pain from occurring in the first place.

What can you do?

One of the best ways to reduce stress is to exercise. Although many people with back trouble may feel that exercise is out of the question, it can not only ease pain, but also improve the health of your back (*see* p. 94). One study claims that regular exercise can reduce stress dramatically. During periods of high stress, those who reported exercising less frequently had 37 per cent more physical symptoms than their counterparts who exercised more often. Exercise works by using up the adrenaline that is created by stress and stressful situations. It also creates endorphins, the 'feel-good' hormones that improve mood, motivation and even tolerance to pain and other stimuli. The best exercise for people with back problems is low-impact aerobic exercise, such as swimming, walking and cycling. And try some of the exercises on pp. 96–105, which work directly on the back itself. **Stretching exercises** can also relieve stress and loosen tight muscles. Yoga (*see* p. 120) incorporates poses that increase strength and flexibility with breathing techniques to relieve stress.

Learn some relaxation techniques (*see* p. 165), which invoke the 'relaxation response'. Muscles relax and blood pressure, heartbeat and respiration decrease. This is the opposite of the 'stress response' where muscles tense and blood pressure, heartbeat and respiration increase. Taking just five minutes a day to relax can have a dramatic impact on your pain.

Massage is also useful for relaxing muscles, increasing circulation and relieving the symptoms of stress (*see* p. 148).

Get proper sleep. Pain can often keep you awake into the early hours, or wake you when you move in your sleep, but there is no doubt that a good night's sleep can help to relieve stress. It helps to be active, to be physically tired at bedtime, so exercise is an important precursor to sleep. Your sleeping position is also important (*see* p. 67), as is your choice of mattress and pillow. Turn on some relaxing music for just five minutes each night to help lull you to sleep. One study found that listening to soothing music as you settle down to sleep resulted in significantly better sleep quality in the experimental group, as well as significantly better components of sleep quality: better perceived sleep quality, longer sleep duration, greater sleep efficiency, less sleep disturbance and less daytime dysfunction.

BACK RELIEF THROUGH POSTURE

One of the simplest and most important ways to keep your back and spine healthy, and to prevent back pain, is to adopt the correct posture – in whatever you may be doing. In fact, studies show that good posture and back support are critical to reducing the incidence of back and neck pain. While you can get away with poor posture for a while, over time the stress you place on your back can lead to constricted blood vessels and nerves, as well problems with the muscles, discs and joints in your back.

In Chapter One we looked at some of the key ways that you can help to maintain the health of your back and prevent injury and pain; here we'll look specifically at how posture – and exercises and positions to encourage good posture – can reduce your pain and strengthen your back.

What is good posture?

Correct posture involves keeping every part of the body in alignment with neighbouring parts – which ensures that everything is both balanced and supported. When you are holding the correct posture while standing, it should be possible to draw a straight line from your earlobe, through your shoulder, hip, knee and into the middle of your ankle. Obviously, however, you don't stand all day, so good posture must be adopted no matter what your activity – sitting, bending, lying down and crouching. It's also important to hold your posture when you switch from one activity or position to another, moving fluidly and smoothly to avoid jerking, abrupt movements and undue pressure on any one part of the body. While this can take some getting used to, these movements will become automatic and require little effort to maintain.

head balanced on top of spine

pressure is exerted on spine as head is pulled back

spine functions well

It's clear to see what happens to the spine when the head goes forwards and up, and when it is pulled back and down.

Standing posture

✔ Stand with weight mostly on the balls of the feet, not with weight on the heels.
✔ Keep feet slightly apart (about shoulder width).
✔ Let arms hang naturally down the sides of the body.
✔ Avoid locking the knees.
✔ Tuck the chin in a little to keep the head level.
✔ Be sure the head is square on top of the neck and spine, not pushed out forward.
✔ Stand straight and tall, with your shoulders upright.

If standing for a long period of time, shift weight from one foot to the other, or rock from heels to toes. Stand against a wall with your shoulders and bottom touching the wall. In this position the back of your head should also touch the wall. If it does not, your head is too far forward.

Walking posture

✔ Keep your head up and eyes looking straight ahead.
✔ Avoid pushing your head forward.
✔ Keep your shoulders properly aligned with the rest of the body.

The Alexander Technique and posture

The Alexander Technique was devised by Australian actor, Frederick Matthias Alexander, who developed problems with his voice. After doctors informed him there was no physical cause, he carefully observed himself with multiple mirrors. This revealed that he was needlessly stiffening his whole body in preparation to recite or speak. It took more than eight years to apply his original observations of himself successfully and solve his voice and performance issues. Eventually, he fashioned a 'technique' to pass on his experiences.

He discovered that the relationship between his head and neck, and how the head and neck relate to the rest of his body, were crucial to correct body use. He called this 'primary control' because this relationship determines the poise and quality of the whole body. He believed that when the head, neck and back work in harmony it contributes to balance in the whole person.

Almost every one of us has effortless poise and balance in childhood. By the time we reach adulthood, however, we've picked up many bad habits of posture and movement. Usually we don't even realise that we have lost our suppleness, because tension has become an unconscious response to stress over a lifetime.

The Alexander Technique addresses these bad habits by helping us to develop an even distribution of muscle tone, neither sloppily relaxed nor overly tense. The philosophy of 'good use' means using and moving the body lightly, with a minimum of interference in the inter-relationship of neck, head and back. The Alexander Technique is a process of re-education, not a 'quick fix solution, although you can use several of the exercises (see pp. 52–9) to make important changes to the way you hold yourself, in some cases instantly relieving even stubborn back pain. Over time, you will find that you function better in almost every way.

A sedentary lifestyle affects posture

The way we move affects our posture, breathing patterns, how we perform our everyday activities and, ultimately, the way we live our lives. A comfortable, easy posture needs a strong and coordinated body. However, a sedentary lifestyle promotes muscle tension. For instance, slumping in a chair for long periods of time compresses the spine. Learning the Alexander Technique can help you to become aware of the inappropriate ways in which you hold, move and use your body, particularly your back. Bad posture and continual muscle misuse can lead to serious musculo-skeletal problems including:

   Head, neck and back pain;
   Muscle aches and spasms;
   Bursitis (inflammation of joints);
   Repetitive strain injuries.

Most of us put too much force into our movements, which can jar nerves, muscles and joints. The Alexander Technique stresses that movement should be 'economical' and needs only the minimum amount of energy and effort. With awareness, it is possible to change postural habits and redistribute muscle effort more evenly and gently throughout the body.

The positioning of your head

'Primary control' – in Alexander's terminology – refers to good 'neuromuscular organisation', which occurs when the whole body is able to expand freely. For this to happen:

✔ The spine must be able to lengthen, which means that the neck must be free;

✔ The head should move in a direction relative to the top of the spine;

✔ The muscles of the back should unclench;

✔ The arms and legs should function as extensions of the back.

Your spine, shoulders and back are thought to be the centrepiece of your body, almost like an imaginary 'cross' that can improve your posture. These remain stable yet supple, creating your centre, and all other joints and muscles are extensions of this strong area. When in a state of natural rest, this area will be balanced and poised, without tension and control. Coordination of the entire body can take place from this centre point. The best way to begin is by making sure your neck is in alignment with your spine, no matter what your stance or activity. This can feel awkward at first, but keeping your eye-level perpendicular to the ground, and your head slightly tipped forward (not craning your neck), will help in the adjustment period. Your head should move smoothly and effortlessly, not rigidly or 'stuck' to your neck.

Becoming aware of how you move

The Alexander Technique focuses on making you aware of how you move and think, no matter what your activity.

Avoid wearing high heels. High-heeled shoes affect good posture because of the way they slant the foot and throw the body out of alignment. Flats with cushioned soles give the best support. The foot is designed to absorb the shock of walking, but with heels the result is a tremendous amount of stress on the back.

Uncross your legs. Crossing your legs, and holding your inner thighs together leads to back problems because of the twist that it creates in the lower back and pelvis. Keeping your legs together as you move can distort the balance between the hip, knee and ankle joints, causing strain. So rather than pulling your knees together after you sit down, keep each knee lined up with your feet. Not ideal for decorum if you are female, but essential for good posture and your back.

Sit straight. It's important to have a chair that supports your lower back and allows your feet to rest comfortably on the floor. If you slouch, your muscles are weakened, ligaments are stretched and there is strain put on the facet joints and discs. When your shoulders slip forward there is also pressure put on your neck. It's important, too, to avoid sitting in odd positions, sitting on one leg, for example, or on a knee. Although it may feel comfortable, it twists your body and does not support your spine. Remember, too, to move around, at least every 20 minutes or so, to prevent the muscles from tiring and tightening.

Bending should be done carefully, without bending at the waist. Your spine has no 'hinge joints' at the waist, so it causes strain on muscles that aren't designed for that kind of work. When you bend, your hips, knees and ankles should do the work.

Try to read at an angle to provide support. On the table, your book should be sloping towards you; in a chair, you can put it on a pillow on your lap to avoid tiring your arms and curving your spine in a slump.

The most important thing is to be aware of your posture. Start paying attention to how you hold yourself. Are your legs relaxed? Is your neck too stiff? Posture should be comfortable.

Sitting comfortably

Try this exercise to improve the way you sit:
Find a chair with good back support, and move your hips to the back of the seat. Try improving your chair design by placing a pillow on the chair back just above the waist to bring you forward and provide thoracic support.

✔ Place your feet flat on the floor or use a footrest.
✔ Without slumping, allow the back of the chair to support you.
✔ Without stiffening, lean into the chair back and envision your back lengthening and widening.
✔ Pay attention to neck and jaw tension. Allow the neck to be free, head poised easily.
✔ Notice your breathing. Allow it to expand to the back and sides of your ribs.
✔ Sit at a comfortable distance from your work surface.
✔ When you look down to read or write, allow your eyes to lower while maintaining the ease of the neck and the poise of the head.
✔ Allow lengthening and widening of the torso. Allow your breath to flow.

Getting help

It is important to take a few classes with a registered Alexander Technique teacher in order to become aware of the poor habits that you have adopted over time. The Alexander Technique is taught using both verbal instructions and the physical guidance of the teacher's hands. It is most often taught in private lessons, although some teachers also work with groups of students. There is no manipulation and no need to remove your clothing. The teacher will help you discover new ways of sitting, standing, breathing and moving that put less pressure on your body and allow you to perform all your daily activities with greater ease and efficiency. The teacher will also demonstrate a new way of thinking about movement, before you actually do it. The more you practise – even in five-minute slots throughout the day – the easier it becomes.

Release your spine in five minutes a day

This position widens and lengthens the spine, helping it to return to its natural alignment, and also encourages the discs to plump up again as they reabsorb the interstitial fluids necessary to maintain the hydraulic pressure in the core of the disc. As well as being vitally important to the back, a few minutes in the semi-supine position can be remarkably calming, restoring and refreshing. A deep level of

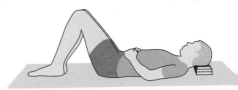

The semi-supine position releases the spine and is good short-term relief for back pain. It helps to lengthen the spine and relieve tension.

physical and psychological repose can be experienced in a short period of time. Try and do it for five minutes every day.

Lay down on the floor with a couple of books under your head (*see* illustration). The pile should be high enough so that your head is not tipping backwards, but not so high that your chin is resting on your chest. Somewhere between the two will bring your head into balance and allow the neck muscles to lengthen.

Move your legs so that they are bent, with your feet flat on the floor, fairly near to your body. Your feet should be shoulder-width apart, so that your legs balance without flopping out to the sides. Equally, however, they should not be held too close together, causing muscle tension. Your knees should point towards the ceiling.

The palms of your hands should be resting on your stomach with your elbows resting on the floor. Slide your legs down again.

Be aware of lying quietly, doing nothing, but focus your attention on the places where your body connects with the floor. Allow the floor to support you.

When it's time to get up, raise your legs up again to a bent position. Gently rock your knees just a little from side to side, then build up some momentum, eventually rolling onto one side and coming onto your hands and knees. Rock a little forward and back a few times, then if possible sit momentarily on your heels. Look down, keep the back of your neck long and calm, and go forward and up to high kneeling. Then bring one foot through in front of you, again look down and keep back of neck long and soft, sending the top of your head forward and up and allowing your body to follow your head into standing. Walk around a little, thinking of your head floating up and out along your spine.

The monkey position

The monkey position – also known as 'the position of mechanical advantage' – encourages maximum balance, openness and muscular release. It is a 'core movement', which most of us lose as we become older, and which needs to be relearnt. Always use this position instead of leaning or bending over.

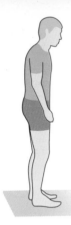
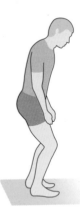

The monkey position is also known as the 'position of mechanical advantage' in the Alexander Technique.

The monkey position is not a still, static position, but a dynamic moving position that you can move in and from. It coordinates the use of the back and legs, a precondition to improving other parts of your body. The 'monkey' is a good way to examine issues of tension, relaxation, balance, posture, position, movement and inhibition. It develops coordination on a general basis, but it is useful whenever you need to lower yourself – to wash your face, brush your teeth, sign a cheque, or pick up an object from the floor.

To go into a 'monkey', stand up and place your feet at shoulder-width or slightly wider apart, pointing your toes outwards slightly.

Bend your knees a little. Now lean forward at the hip joint.

Check frequently that you're 'hinge-ing' correctly at the hip joints, not in the lower back. When you first bend your knees, don't let your chest drop forwards and don't stick your bottom out behind you. You should stay upright, undisturbed by the bending of your knees. Take care, too, not to tighten your toes or stiffen your arms. When you lean forward, your head should lead and your body should follow. Don't slump or hollow your back – allow your spine to lengthen and widen as you move.

The 'monkey' in childbirth

The 'monkey' is one of the best positions to use during pregnancy and is particularly advantageous during labour. As you lean forward, your abdominal wall becomes a kind of hammock for the baby, while the tilt of your pelvis makes more space for the baby's head to enter the pelvic brim; thus the baby is encouraged to move into the optimal position for birth. At the same time, the force of gravity – the weight of the baby – aids contractions and makes them stronger and more efficient.

Back against the wall

This could loosely be described as an exercise (although this was a term that Alexander hated) as it involves a little movement (a very slow bending and unbending of the legs from a standing position). The aim is to encourage lengthening and widening of the spine while upright. When we stand, our spines lapse into a curve as a response to gravity, and over time we develop bad habits or 'patterns of misuse'. Stand with your feet about 15 cm (6 in) from a wall, hip-width apart or wider. Lean back against the wall. Your knees should be nearly straight, but not locked. Your head should be poised on your neck, free of the

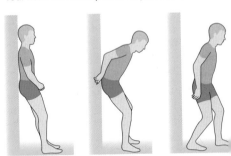

The back against the wall exercise is adapted in this illustration to show how gentle movements can help reduce back pain.

wall. Imagine your body lengthening and widening. Notice your breathing. If your back is tight, bend your knees slightly and focus on releasing tension in both the back and neck. Gently bend your knees and rise.

This simple yet effective position and gentle movement can be used as the basis for other exercises. The following will help with lower back pain: Put yourself in the back-against-the-wall position.

✔ Gently anchor your shoulder blades against the wall.

✔ Tuck your chin against your chest and then release it slowly – 'relaxing' your head and neck forward and away from the wall. There should be no movement, just a feeling of release.

✔ Push the small of your back into the wall and then breathe normally. Allow your neck to be free, with your head forward and up. Without changing the shape of your spine, neck or head, lean forward.

✔ Slowly push yourself up and away from the wall and start walking with your feet flat on the floor. Keep the small of your back in the position that it was against the wall, and make sure your head is comfortably loose on your neck – forward and up.

Everyday posture

Being 'mindful' of the way you hold yourself as you go about your daily tasks and activities can make a big difference to your posture and, through that, your back problems.

BACK RELIEF THROUGH IMPROVED NUTRITION

You may be surprised to learn that your diet and the nutrients it contains can have a big effect on the health of your back and the pain you experience. Your bones, muscles and the other structures in your spine require good nutrition in order to be strong enough to support the body and perform their other functions. Let's look at what a healthy back needs.

Calcium

This mineral is essential for healthy, strong bones and it may help to prevent the onset of osteoporosis, a condition in which the bones (including those of the spine) become weak and brittle. The best sources of calcium include: dairy produce, broccoli, kale and other leafy green vegetables, soya, peanuts, peas, baked beans, sesame seeds, almonds, brown sugar and salmon.

Vitamin D

Known as the 'sunshine vitamin', this regulates blood levels of calcium and phosphorus, and is required for bones to absorb calcium. Your body is able to make its own vitamin D in the presence of sunlight; food sources include milk, salmon and tuna.

Manganese

Manganese is a trace mineral that is beneficial for bone metabolism and growth. Good sources include beetroot, broccoli, barley, rice, oats, sunflower seeds, tofu, raspberries, walnuts, quinoa, almonds, chocolate, blueberries and sweet potatoes.

Vitamin B12

One of the important B vitamins, this one in particular is necessary for healthy bone marrow and for the body (including the spine) to grow and function normally. B vitamins are important for a healthy nervous system, too. You'll find B12 in meat products, fish, dairy produce, eggs and leafy green vegetables.

Vitamin C

This is one of the 'antioxidant' nutrients (*see* p. 63) and it is necessary for the development of collagen, which is an important part of the process that allows cells to be able to form into tissue. This is extremely important for healing problems caused by injured tendons, ligaments and vertebral discs, as well as for keeping bones and other tissues strong. Brightly coloured fruits and vegetables contain good levels of vitamin C, as do potatoes (both sweet and white).

Vitamin A

Another antioxidant, this vitamin is great for backs because it helps to repair tissue and is important in forming bone. You'll find it in dairy produce, eggs and beef. Beta carotene is a compound related to vitamin A, and the body can convert it into vitamin A. It's found in brightly coloured fruits and vegetables. Carrots, spinach, sweet potatoes, apricots and nectarines are excellent sources.

Magnesium

This mineral is important for the relaxing and contracting of muscles. It also helps maintain muscle tone and bone density, which in turn can help prevent back problems. Look for it in whole grains, beans, seeds, nuts, avocados, bananas, kiwi and leafy green vegetables.

Some extra help

Bromelain is an enzyme found in pineapple, and several studies show that it can ease the aching and stiffness of back muscles.

EFAs (essential fatty acids) are the omega oils you've probably read plenty about. They are found in fish oils and hemp (flaxseed oil), as well as quinoa, fresh fatty fish (such as salmon or mackerel), raw nuts and seeds, and unsaturated vegetable oils. EFAs are crucial for health (which explains why they are called essential) on all levels, and every cell in the body requires them for rebuilding and renewal. What's more, they are used by the body in the production of hormone-like substances called prostaglandins, which have many uses, including acting as anti-inflammatory agents. A 2006 study found that fish oils were as (if not more) effective as anti-inflammatory medications, such as ibuprofen, in the treatment of back pain. Some 60 per cent of respondents reported significant improvement, including reduction in overall pain, and 59 per cent were able to stop taking pain medication.

Antioxidant nutrients (vitamins A, C and E, plus the minerals selenium and zinc) are known to slow down the degenerative effects of ageing, which can be crucial not only as we age, but as the body begins to show signs of 'wear and tear'. Nuts, seeds and brightly coloured fruits and vegetables are good sources, as are whole grains and shellfish.

BACK RELIEF IN THE BEDROOM

Sleep is often difficult for many people with back pain, as the discomfort can make falling asleep difficult, and any movements in the night excruciating. A good mattress and pillow can make a big difference, as can adopting a healthy position for sleeping and for sex. Getting in and out of bed correctly will also help to ensure that any problems are not exacerbated. For morning stiffness or tenderness, try a few simple exercises to get you on your feet with the minimum of pain.

Your mattress

A mattress that does not offer enough support for your spine can lead to muscle fatigue and a poor night's sleep. A good mattress will allow you to maintain the same natural spinal alignment that you have when standing. When your body is allowed to rest in its natural position, muscles are relaxed and sleep is more refreshing.

Many mattress manufacturers promote extra-firm surfaces, but it is possible for a mattress to be too firm. Similarly, some mattresses may be too soft, especially ones that come with extra soft feather tops. Neither situation allows your muscles to rest, as they must work through the night to find a comfortable position and maintain correct posture.

Because back pain is individual to the sufferer, as are sleeping positions and even body shape and size, there is no 'best' mattress for back pain. You'll need to choose one that feels comfortable, while offering support. Having said that, a recent study found that medium-firm mattresses provide the best support for back-pain sufferers. The reason for this is that a too-firm mattress can cause pain and aching at pressure points, while one that is medium-firm allows the shoulders and hips to sink in slightly.

If your current mattress is too hard, you can purchase padding to put over the top. Similarly, a mattress that is too soft can be underlaid with a board.

Make sure your mattress is still doing the job. If it sags in the middle, it's time for a replacement. Similarly, if you find you are not sleeping comfortably, you may need to change to a different type of mattress. Studies show that mattresses on box springs (divans) provide the best support, rather than being set directly on the slats of the bed. Furthermore, it's a good idea to flip and turn your mattress every six months to ensure that it is evenly worn.

Some people find that an adjustable bed helps to ease pain and promote good sleep. The idea is that the head of the bed can be slightly raised (no more than 45 degrees) and, with additional support under the knees, can help reduce pain, particularly that caused by disc problems or spinal stenosis (*see* pp. 13–14). It also makes it easier to get into and out of bed without having to roll or sit up.

A water bed may also be appropriate, as it distributes body weight more evenly than do other types of mattresses. A good rule of thumb is to use whatever is most comfortable for you.

Pillows

In addition to providing comfort, the right pillows can also provide the necessary support for the neck and spine, alleviating or preventing many common forms of back and neck pain.

Choose a pillow that keeps your spine in natural alignment. Our necks naturally curve slightly forward, to sustain the weight of our heads when they are upright, and this curve should be maintained in sleep. If your pillow is too high (whether you are sleeping on your back or your side), your neck will be bent abnormally, causing muscle strain. A pillow that is too low in height will, paradoxically, do the same. The ideal pillow is about 10–15 cm (4–6 in) in height, and it should support your head and neck when lying on your back.

Your pillow should also be comfortable. Ideally, it should mould to your individual shape and alleviate any pressure points. Unless they are well stuffed, most down or feather pillows offer very little structural support compared to pillows filled with firmer materials. People who suffer from back or neck pain, and, in particular disc problems, seem to experience a more restful night's sleep with a firmer pillow. When your pillow is no longer firm and holding its shape, it should be replaced.

Sleeping positions

Certain sleeping positions can trigger back pain by throwing the spine out of alignment and by unduly stretching the back muscles. Lying on your stomach, particularly with a pillow under your head, stresses the neck and exaggerates the curve of the lower back.

The best sleeping positions for people with back discomfort are those that maintain the natural curves of the spine. Here are some suggestions:

Sleep on your side with your knees slightly tucked up (a light 'foetal' position); this position puts the least strain on your back. A pillow between your knees reduces the pressure even more.

If you prefer to sleep on your back, use a pillow under your knees and your head/neck.

Sleeping on your stomach will put the spine into an unnatural position and can lead directly to morning backache. If it's the only way that you can sleep, try putting a pillow under your tummy but nothing under your head.

Getting in and out of bed

As you are lying on your back, roll over onto your side so you are facing the side of the bed you plan to get out of. Gently bring your knees toward your chest, keeping your legs in contact with the bed at all times. As you do this, simultaneously use your hands and arms to push your upper body up off of the bed; let your legs fall slowly off of the edge. As your upper body raises up, most of your weight will be on the hip, buttocks and thighs rather than on the spine. Complete the manoeuvre by putting your hands on your thighs and extending your back up as you push yourself up and out of bed. Keep your back straight and your head up as you rise. There

Take your time getting out of bed, placing both feet together before gently swinging them to the floor and rolling off.

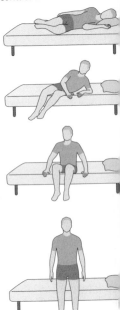

should be a rolling movement at all times, never any jerking or twisting. Take your time, particularly in the morning, as backs often 'go' first thing because they haven't 'warmed up'.

Remember, getting back into bed can also be stressful, even to a healthy back. It can be tempting to flop into bed at the end of the day, but the forced twisting that such a fall can cause is dangerous. Use this technique in reverse to get into bed – moving slowly, and rolling rather than twisting.

Five-minute exercises to relieve pain

These are great exercises to warm up your back before you try to get out of bed. Not only will you reduce morning stiffness that may cause pain or potentially injure your back, but you will also relieve any pain caused by congestion while you sleep.

Exercise One

Lie on your back. Place a small pillow under your head and one or two large pillows under your knees. For five minutes concentrate on relaxing your back muscles, starting from the base of your spine up to your shoulders and neck, and then down again. Lightly flex and release your neck, shoulders and spine.

Exercise Two

Remove the pillows from under your knees, but keep your knees bent. Now gently pull your legs (one at a time) to your chest. Hold for a few seconds. Do this three times for each leg. Then repeat the process doing both legs at the same time.

Bedtime play

Sex is often one of the first activities to be sidelined when you suffer from back pain; however, it's worth remembering that the benefits can be significant. For one thing, sex is a gentle form of exercise and it is known to lift mood and improve self-image. Many back-pain sufferers feel dreadful about themselves and their loss of mobility and, in some cases, their inability to do normal things plays havoc with their self-esteem. Pain can make people irritable, and a lack of physical contact and touch can strain even the best relationships. Becoming close to your partner can help you to feel good about yourself and maintain important closeness.

There are a number of sexual positions that should not cause any discomfort; but it's important to remember that you should stop the moment that things become painful. Adopting a new position should ease things tremendously. Try:

The missionary position. *Women with back trouble:* Keep your knees bent to relieve stress on your lower back. Lie on a firm surface and place a rolled towel under your lower back and/or your knees, to keep them flexed. *Men with back trouble:* This can be a difficult position to adopt, as thrusting or holding yourself upon your forearms can be tiring and painful. Best to avoid this position.

Spoons. This position works for either partner with back problems. Lie on your side and put a pillow between your knees. Enter from the rear, curving your body around your partner. It may help to keep your head on a shared pillow to give you both more support.

Sitting. This is a good position if either of you has back pain, as it gives you some control over the position of your back. *Women with back trouble:* Sit on your partner's lap and experiment a bit with comfortable positions. Use the back of the chair or the head of the bed to distribute your weight and for extra support. Alternatively, kneel over your sitting partner and support your weight on your elbows. *Men with back problems:* Lie on your back with your lower back and knees supported by towels or pillows. Your partner can straddle you in the kneeling position; you also might like to try this in a chair.

Whatever you choose, be gentle and respectful if your partner is uncomfortable. Sometimes just a tiny shift in position can make a difference. Use as many 'props' as required – offering support to your back, knees and neck with pillows or rolled-up towels can make all the difference.

BACK RELIEF DURING PREGNANCY, LABOUR AND BEYOND

Between 50 and 80 per cent of women experience some back pain during pregnancy, ranging from mild pain associated with specific activities to acute back pain that can become chronic. Studies show that low back pain usually occurs between the fifth and seventh months of pregnancy, but can begin as early as eight to twelve weeks into pregnancy. Women with pre-existing lower back problems are at higher risk for back pain, and their back pain can occur earlier in the pregnancy.

There are a number of common causes. Weight gain is an obvious one – extra pounds add stress to your back and the weight-bearing structures that surround them. Second, your centre of gravity changes as weight shifts to the front of your body, causing muscular imbalances and fatigue. This in turn can create poor posture and exacerbate existing problems (such as muscle weakness or inflexibility, or even previous strains or injuries). Pregnancy hormones also cause problems by loosening the ligaments and other supporting structures to prepare the body for childbirth – this means that the joints become lax and there is less support.

What's more, ligaments, muscles, discs and joints can be placed under strain from poor posture, bad lifting technique, weak or tight muscles or injury. Back pain often gets worse towards the end of the day or if you have been on your feet for a long time. This is due to your muscles becoming tired and your ligaments stretching slightly from the weight of your body and baby.

Some women suffer from sciatica (*see* p. 13) during pregnancy. This is not caused by your baby pressing on the sciatic nerve, but is the result of inflammation and/or pressure from the structures of the back affecting the nerve. There are two other conditions that may cause back pain, both of which need to be seen by a specialist, as regular back-pain treatment can be ineffective and even make these conditions worse. One is pelvic girdle pain and the other is symphysis pubis dysfunction, where pain is experienced around the pubic bone at the front. For this reason, any back pain during pregnancy should be reported to your doctor.

Five-minute tips for pregnancy back pain

Ask your partner for a five-minute massage (*see* p. 155). Try leaning forward over the back of a chair or lying on your side; the muscles that run on either side of the spine and across the lower back should be the focus.

Purchase a support belt. These are designed to take some of the weight of your baby off your abdominal muscles and back.

Try kneeling on your hands and knees. This is an excellent position for reducing pressure on your back from the weight of your baby and you should attempt to adopt this position regularly throughout the day. Try rounding your back up into a hump shape (tucking your tailbone underneath you) and then gently arching your back in the opposite direction so that you stick your bottom out (this movement is sometimes known as 'humping and hollowing'). Repeating this in a rocking motion can be very useful for back or pelvic pain.

Pelvic floor exercises and lower abdominal exercises can help to reduce the strain of the pregnancy on your back. To perform a safe and easy lower abdominal exercise, get down onto your hands and knees and after 'humping and hollowing' (see above), level your back so that it is roughly flat. Breathe in and then, as you breathe out, perform a pelvic floor exercise (see opposite) and at the same time pull your belly button in and up. Hold this for five to ten seconds without holding your breath and without moving your back. Relax the muscles slowly at the end of the exercise.

Pelvic floor exercises (kegels) are essential. The pelvic floor muscles form a broad sling between your legs from the pubic bone in front to the base of your spine at the back. They help to hold the bladder, womb and bowel in place and to control the muscles that close the anus, vagina and urethra. Pressure on these muscles during pregnancy and childbirth can weaken them, making the muscles less effective and putting pressure on other supporting muscles and ligaments. Pelvic floor exercises can strengthen these muscles so that they function effectively again. The more you use them, the stronger they will be. Strong pelvic floor muscles can support the extra weight of pregnancy and help in the second stage of labour.

Performing pelvic floor exercises

1. Begin by emptying your bladder.

2. Tighten the pelvic floor muscles. (If you have trouble finding them, try stopping and starting the flow of urine when you are on the toilet. These are the muscles you want to work.) Hold for a count of ten.

3. Relax the muscle completely for a count of ten.

4. Perform ten exercises, three times a day (morning, afternoon and night).

These exercises can be performed any time and any place. Most people prefer to perform the exercises while lying down or sitting in a chair. Just five minutes, three times a day can make a big difference.

Pelvic tilting can help to minimise the strain placed on your back by prolonged standing.

Stand with your back against a wall. Position your feet a few centimetres away from the wall and allow your knees to bend very slightly. Slide your hand into the hollow of your back and tilt your pelvis backwards so that your back squashes your hand. Now tilt your pelvis the opposite way so that the pressure from your back is removed from your hand. Continue to tilt forwards and backwards in a rhythmical fashion. Once you are confident with this exercise, you can perform it away from the wall.

Pilates exercises (see pp. 108–119) are based on movement patterns performed with your tummy and pelvic floor muscles – known as the 'stable core' or base. These muscles are also known as deep stabilising muscles, and they can weaken during pregnancy. Pilates exercises, which target these muscles, can be useful. Many Pilates exercises are performed in a 'hands and knees' position, which is an ideal position for pregnancy. It helps take a lot of stress off your back and pelvis, and towards the end of your pregnancy can help to position your baby ready for delivery.

The best childbirth positions

Labour itself can put enormous pressure on the back and supporting structure, and the position of your baby in the pelvis can also make things worse. For example, a posterior labour (where the baby's spine is against yours instead of facing outwards) can cause tremendous discomfort. In all cases you'll need to find a position that feels comfortable, and which takes the strain off your back.

Standing is a good one, particularly if you adopt the monkey position (*see* pp. 55–7) and lean forward slightly onto your partner or the back of a chair. This helps speed up labour because it enlists the help of gravity and takes the pressure off your back, while aligning the baby with your pelvic angle.

Sitting upright with full support behind your back also encourages a quicker birth, particularly if you are able to sit cross-legged (which opens the pelvis).

Kneeling on your hands and knees can help to relieve back pain, and may also work to rotate a posterior baby. It can be tiring, but you can prop yourself up with beanbags and cushions to take the pressure off your arms.

Avoid semi-sitting, which increases back pain. Similarly, lying on your side may be an excellent resting position, but it slows down the labour, which may exacerbate pain and back problems.

Lying on your back is the worst position for back pain. Not only is it the least effective position for the progress of labour, but it will increase backache significantly.

During the second stage, lying at a 45-degree angle is much better than lying flat, but make sure you pull up your knees and elevate your back and shoulders firmly. Some women prefer to lie on their sides, which is also good for backache, and makes it easier to relax between pushes. If you aren't already exhausted, the best position for delivery is on your hands and knees, as the pressure switches to the abdominal muscles and legs rather than the back structures.

Coping with your new baby

For several weeks and even months after the birth, your weakened ligaments and other supporting structures will make injury more likely. What's more, any strain or injury caused during pregnancy or labour will take some time to heal, and you may find that your postpartum back pain is significant.

At this time, it's extremely important to adopt all of the golden rules for back care (see p. 28–37), taking care to lift, sit, hold your posture, bend and sleep correctly. Also consider the following:

Avoid heavy lifting. As your ligaments are more pliable, you may be more vulnerable to injury. If you have to lift or carry anything, hold it close to your body, bend your knees rather than your back (as if squatting) and try not to twist.

If you have a toddler or small child to care for as well, ask them to climb onto a chair or sofa before you pick them up. Try to encourage more mobile, older toddlers to climb into their car seats or high chairs themselves.

When shopping, divide your purchases into two equal loads and carry one bag in each hand.

Watch the weight of your baby bag. Just take the essentials when you go out, and change the shoulder or arm you are using for carrying regularly.

Begin gentle exercise soon after delivery to restore muscle tone to the abdominal and back muscles. While the baby is napping, take five minutes to do stretching exercises on the floor each day. This will help restore hip and back flexibility.

Do not stretch out your arms when you pick up your baby. Bring the baby close to your chest before lifting, and avoid any twisting.

When you pick up your baby from the floor, bend at your knees, not at your waist, and squat down. Tighten your abdominal muscles and lift with your legs.

Remove the high chair tray when you are trying to put your baby in or out of the high chair.

Make sure that your changing table is at waist height or slightly higher, so that you do not have to crouch over to deal with nappies. Similarly, use a raised surface to bathe your new baby in a baby bath. Even the kitchen sink lined with flannels, or a clean washing-up bowl, is a better choice than bending over a bathtub.

When you lift your baby out of a cot, put down the side and pull the baby towards you, avoiding bending and lifting.

There has been considerable debate about the various merits of front and back carriers and their potential to cause back pain, and it seems that the jury is still out. Experts recommend that either is acceptable, as long as the shoulder straps are snug, it has a waist strap as well as shoulder straps (to prevent too much pressure on any one part of the body) and it holds your baby high up on your body, above the waist and stomach.

Avoid carrying your baby on your hip without support, as this overloads the back muscles and causes contortion. Having said that, when your baby is old enough (from six months), consider investing in a hip seat (a back-supporting belt with an integral padded foam shelf), developed to allow adults to carry their children naturally on their hip without the usual strains on the back. The seat provides a firm shelf for the child to sit on and supports their increasingly heavy weight from underneath. Instead of twisting the spine, the back stays straight and the child is tucked into the chest on the side that is more comfortable for the wearer.

To avoid upper back pain from breastfeeding, bring your baby to your breast, rather than bending over to the baby. While you are nursing, sit in an upright chair rather than a soft couch. Place a pillow under your baby to lift them to your breast, or consider feeding lying down on your side, with an arm cradled under your baby's head.

MEDICAL HELP FOR BACK RELIEF

Apart from medication (*see* pp. 22–4), your doctor may suggest other therapies or treatments both to ease your pain and to encourage healing of any trauma causing the pain. Doctors follow guidelines based on clinical knowledge and procedure, so you can expect to be treated according to a series of directives.

The National Institute for Health and Clinical Excellence (NICE) is an independent organisation responsible for providing national guidance on the promotion of good health and the prevention and treatment of ill health. Guidance for non-specific lower back pain is at present being commissioned and is due in 2009. However, there is a draft document available. This outlines the aims of the therapies available and the ways that doctors can and should manage the use of medication, exercise therapies, manual therapies, physical therapies and referrals for surgery. It also describes how they can implement lifestyle interventions, such as patient education and advice, workplace interventions and pain management through psychological means.

In Chapter One we looked at the causes of back pain, as well as the various means of identifying them. Treatment options will vary according to your individual characteristics, overall health, age and the cause of your problems. Here we'll look in detail at some of the treatments your doctor might suggest, such as neurostimulation, as well as using heat and cold to reduce pain and encourage healing.

The treatments described on pp. 83–6 represent an emerging area of study. As new information becomes available changes in the application of these techniques for treatment may be necessary. The reader is advised to consult their practitioner before embarking on any of these methods of treatment.

BACK RELIEF THROUGH ELECTRICAL STIMULATION

Electrical techniques, such as neurostimulation, deliver low-voltage electrical stimulation to a targeted nerve, muscle or spinal cord to block the sensation of pain. First used in the 1960s, electrical stimulation of the peripheral nerves was shown to mask pain with a tingling sensation (paraesthesia). This mechanism is part of the gate control theory of pain, proposing that a gate exists in the spinal cord that controls the transmission of pain signals to the brain. A variety of different electrical techniques are now used to mask pain.

TENS

A procedure called transcutaneous electrical nerve stimulation (TENS) uses a battery-operated unit to send a weak electrical current through specific points on the skin to nerve pathways. This is believed to interrupt pain signals, preventing them from reaching your brain. Although safe and painless, TENS doesn't work for everyone or for all types of pain. It's generally more effective for acute pain than for chronic pain and is often used with other treatments. TENS may be a good option to try for people who can't take or don't get relief from medication. The advantage of TENS is that you can use your unit at home, and control the stimulation according to the pain you are experiencing, putting you in charge of your own pain relief. Electrodes can be placed over the painful area, surrounding the painful area, over the nerve supplying the painful area, or even on the opposite side of the body.

IFC

Interferential current (IFC) is essentially a deeper form of TENS. Tiny electrical impulses are delivered to the area of the pain. Where these waves intersect below the surface of the skin, the stimulation creates a pain block or leads to the secretion of endorphins, your body's natural painkillers. Interferential current is used for the symptomatic relief and management of chronic, intractable pain and for post-surgical and post-injury acute pain.

GS

If your back pain has become severe, you might think about Galvanic Stimulation. This is thought to be most useful in acute injuries associated with major tissue trauma with bleeding or swelling. In contrast to TENS and IFC units, which apply alternating current, galvanic stimulators apply a direct current. The direct current creates an electrical field over the treated area which, theoretically, changes blood flow.

The positive pad behaves like ice, causing reduced circulation to the area under the pad and reduction in swelling. The negative pad behaves like heat, causing increased circulation and, reportedly, speeding healing.

ALTENS and ETPS

In this technique, strong electrical stimulation is applied through needles placed beneath the skin. It is referred to as Electroacupuncture or Acupuncture

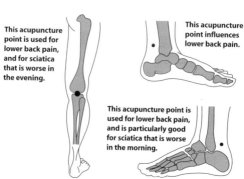

This acupuncture point is used for lower back pain, and for sciatica that is worse in the evening.

This acupuncture point influences lower back pain.

This acupuncture point is used for lower back pain, and is particularly good for sciatica that is worse in the morning.

Electro Therapeutic Point Stimulation (ETPS) involves applying electrical stimulation to the skin at acupuncture points with a hand-held instrument, in order to reduce and even eradicate pain.

Like Transcutaneous Nerve Stimulation (ALTENS). It is used to optimise the release of endorphins (natural painkillers) to combat pain. Electro Therapeutic Point Stimulation (ETPS) is a new therapy for chronic and acute pain. It is a non-invasive therapy applying low-frequency electrical stimulation to the skin at acupuncture points, motor/trigger points and contracted motor bands (that is, bands of muscles that are tense or 'contracted'). ETPS is based upon the premise that ancient philosophies combined with modern electrotherapy technology can provide therapeutic results to suffering patients. Patients are given a hand-held instrument. It takes about a day to learn how to use it to alleviate and even eliminate your own pain. One study found that over 75 per cent of patients with difficult (chronic) pain problems using ETPS had at least 50 per cent relief after one five-minute treatment.

BACK RELIEF THROUGH PHYSIOTHERAPY

Many doctors will refer you to a physiotherapist for both acute and chronic back pain. In the UK you are now able to self-refer as well, which means going directly to a physiotherapist for treatment, without seeing your GP first.

A physiotherapist can apply a variety of treatments such as heat, ice, ultrasound, electrical stimulation and muscle-release techniques to your back muscles and soft tissues to reduce pain. As pain lessens, the therapist can teach you specific exercises to increase your flexibility, strengthen your back and abdominal muscles, and improve your posture. Regular use of these techniques is believed to help pain from recurring.

Many therapists use a series of exercises with a Swiss ball (also known as a physio ball) to help prevent further episodes of low back pain as part of a rehabilitation programme. The exercise ball is effective in rehabilitating the back because it helps strengthen and develop the core body muscles that help to stabilise the spine. In addition, it is believed that the type of spinal movement induced by using the exercise ball (small range, adjustment of balance) may help reduce pain by stimulating the body to produce increased amounts of natural pain inhibitors –

the endorphins. You'll find some good exercises using a Swiss ball on pp.103–6.

Physiotherapy is not as widely used in the UK as it is in the US and, in particular, New Zealand (where 48 per cent of back-pain sufferers are referred, compared with only 12 per cent in the UK), and its benefits have been questioned. For example, a 2004 study found that routine physiotherapy for mild back pain is no more effective than a single advice session about how to remain active.

GPR

Many physiotherapists are now using an innovative technique that may relieve back pain even when all other treatments fail. The technique, called Souchard's global postural re-education (GPR), consists of a series of gentle movements to realign spinal column joints and strengthen and stretch muscles that have become tight and weak from underuse. The idea is to take pressure off of the spinal cord. One study found that nine in ten people with chronic back pain due to disc disease significantly improved and were able to return to their usual daily activities, usually within five months. Developed in France, GPR is now practised by many physiotherapists in Europe, Australia and the US.

BACK RELIEF THROUGH HEAT

Many episodes of back pain result from strains and over-exertion, creating tension in the muscles and soft tissues around the lower spine. As a result, this restricts proper circulation and sends pain signals to the brain. Heat therapy can help relieve pain from muscle spasm and related tightness in the lower back.

Heat therapy works in a number of ways:

Heat dilates the blood vessels of the muscles surrounding the spine. This process increases the flow of oxygen and nutrients to the muscles, helping to heal the damaged tissue.

Heat stimulates the sensory receptors in the skin, so applying heat to the painful area will decrease transmissions of pain signals to the brain and partially relieve the discomfort.

Heat encourages the soft tissues around the spine, including muscles, connective tissue and adhesions, to stretch. Therefore, any stiffness should be relieved with the increase in flexibility.

One of the main benefits of heat therapy is that it can be undertaken at home. A hot bath, for example, can make a significant difference to both pain and mobility; portable heat wraps can be used in your car, at home when relaxing, or at work. For most people, heat therapy works best when you combine it with other treatments, such as stretching and gentle exercise.

Self-help heat therapy

Remember first that heat therapy does not mean boiling hot therapy. Warm is the correct temperature, allowing heat to penetrate down into the muscles without burning the skin.

In some cases you will need to keep your heat source on for longer than five or ten minutes, particularly at the outset. However, for minor back tension and regularly heat-treated muscles, a short period is enough. Just repeat several times a day as required.

Dry-heat options include electric heating pads and saunas. These can be used for just a few minutes a day to warm the back muscles and the surrounding area for instant relief.

Moist heat such as hot baths, steamed towels or moist heating packs can encourage the heat to penetrate into the muscles and some people feel that moist heat provides better pain relief. A steam bath, which produces wet heat, is also suitable.

Try a hot water bottle wrapped in a moist towel, or a heated gel pack, which is normally microwaved or heated in water. Wrap in a warm, damp towel and when it cools, remove to benefit directly from the heat of the gel pack.

Heat wraps are normally used around the lower back and waist and may be worn against the skin under your clothing. These take only a few minutes to prepare and offer several hours of warmth. Hot baths, whirlpools or hot tubs encourage general relaxation, which can reduce muscle spasm and pain. You can direct the jets of a whirlpool directly onto the affected area to reduce pain. Just a few minutes is long enough to have an affect on pain.

Keeping warm

Cold muscles are more susceptible to strain and injury because they are not as flexible. Muscle elasticity depends on how much blood is running through them, so cold muscles with little blood in them are more likely to become injured or damaged. Therefore, it is important to keep them warm at all times. In practice, this means:

✔ Covering up in clothing that keeps your back warm. This doesn't mean tight clothing that will prevent blood flow to the area, but keeping warm, particularly when it is cold outside.

✔ Warm up carefully before exercise. Once again, you must get the blood flowing through the muscles. Even on a hot day, your muscles may not be warm enough to provide full flexibility.

✔ Don't assume that warming sprays, gels or creams will warm your muscles. In many cases they work only on the skin and the surface areas of the muscles and ligaments, not warming them deeply enough to prevent injury or strain.

✔ Heated car seats or portable heated car-seat cushions are a good bet. Not only do they keep the blood supply active when you are driving, preventing stiffness and problems associated with cold muscles, but they also relax the muscles, thereby reducing pain. Portable cushions can be used on trains, buses, airplanes or at home, as well as in your car. You can also find heating pads that will plug into the cigarette lighter in your car.

✔ If you sleep in a cool room at night, try using a heating pad or regular electric blanket under your bottom sheet (don't forget to switch it off after use) to keep your back warm and supple.

Warning

Heat should not be used in certain circumstances. For example, if the lower back is swollen or bruised, it is better to use a cold pack to reduce the inflammation or swelling in the area. You should also check with your doctor if you have heart disease or hypertension. In general, heat therapy should also not be used if you suffer from dermatitis, deep vein thrombosis, diabetes, peripheral vascular disease, an open wound or severe cognitive impairment.

What about ice?

While heat is used to keep your muscles warm and flexible, ice is used to decrease the swelling associated with inflammation. To relieve initial pain and swelling, apply ice packs or bags of frozen vegetables wrapped in towels for five to ten minutes every two hours for the first two days, and then apply heat or ice as needed.

Ice massage and ice application are generally most helpful during the first 48 hours following an injury that strains the back muscles. After this initial period, heat therapy is probably more beneficial to the healing process because it encourages the flow of blood and oxygen to the area. For some people, alternating heat therapy with cold applications such as ice massage therapy (*see* p. 157) provides the most pain relief.

BACK RELIEF THROUGH EXERCISE

Exercise is the single most important element of any programme undertaken to protect your back, relieve pain, prevent further injury and encourage a positive frame of mind – now known to be an important factor in pain of all descriptions. All doctors recommend gentle exercise, and this forms the central advice given to every back-pain sufferer by physiotherapists, medical practitioners and alternative therapists.

There are countless ways that exercise can help your back: general exercises to improve mobility, strength and flexibility, including McKenzie exercises (see pp. 99–103), stretching exercises, yoga, Pilates, water-based exercises such as swimming and aquarobics, and even just walking. In most cases few, if any, props are required and most can be highly effective – in some cases with a little advance training – in just a few minutes a day. In this chapter we'll look at what is available, how to practise the exercises, which exercises can be used for instant pain relief and long-term benefit, and how to fit them into a busy day.

Why exercise?

Gentle, gradual exercise slowly built up into a regular programme over time plays an important role in dealing with back problems. For one thing, exercise improves the circulation, which distributes oxygen and nutrients into the disc space and soft tissues of your back, keeping the discs, muscles, ligaments and joints healthy. This also prevents weakness and stiffness, and reduces the severity of future episodes of pain. Exercise also reduces muscle spasm and encourages the release of natural painkillers, called endorphins, as well as lifting mood and overall well-being. A good exercise programme should include active exercise (low-impact aerobics, for example), stretching, strengthening and conditioning.

GENERAL EXERCISES

All of the following exercises can be undertaken at home, and are recommended by doctors and specialists. It's a good idea to speak to your doctor before undertaking any exercise programme. While all of these exercises are simple to follow and enhance the health of your back, some conditions may preclude their use.

This section contains basic exercises to strengthen or improve the flexibility of your back. Before every exercise, take care to warm up by doing some gentle stretching (see p. 100); following exercise, stretch again to warm down. Drink plenty of water during any exercise programme to ensure that you are well hydrated; back pain is often caused by dehydration, according to various studies.

The best exercise for backs

Apart from single exercises, which can be done in short bursts, or spread throughout the day, it is also important to undertake exercise that improves your overall health – your circulation, heart, lungs and muscles. In most cases, this involves aerobic exercise (see pp. 130–39), for about 20 minutes every day.

Five-minute strengthening exercises

These work on the muscles of your back, legs, buttocks and hips, to make them stronger and more flexible.

Wall slides

These strengthen your back, hip and leg muscles.

Stand with your back against a wall and feet shoulder-width apart. Slide down into a crouch with your knees bent to about 90 degrees. Count to five and slide back up the wall. Repeat five times.

Leg raises

Leg raises strengthen your back and hip muscles.

Lie on your stomach. Tighten the muscles in one leg and raise it from the floor. Hold your leg up for a count of ten and return it to the floor. Do the same with the other leg. Repeat five times with each leg.

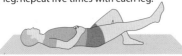

Leg raises can help with the pain of sciatica.

Chair raises

This exercise strengthens stomach and hip muscles.

Sit upright in a chair with your legs straight and extended at an angle to the floor. Lift one leg to waist height. Slowly return your leg to the floor. Do the same with the other leg. Repeat the exercise five times with each leg.

Exercise to decrease the strain on your back

Lie on your back with your knees bent and feet flat on the floor. Raise your knees towards your chest. Place both hands under your knees and gently pull your knees as close to your chest as possible. Do not raise your head. Lower your legs with your knees bent (do not straighten them). Repeat five times.

Abdominal contractions

This exercise works to strengthen your abdominal muscles, which help to support the back and spine.

Lie on your back with your knees bent and your hands resting just below your ribs. Tighten your abdominal muscles to 'squeeze' your ribs down toward your back. Continue to breathe normally throughout (no breath-holding allowed!). Hold for five seconds and relax. Repeat five times.

Knee-to-chest stretch

Lie on your back with both of your knees bent. Hold your thigh behind one knee and bring it up to your chest. Hold this position for 20 seconds and then relax. Repeat five times on each side.

McKenzie exercises

McKenzie exercises, named after a physiotherapist in New Zealand, work by extending the spine to reduce the pressure on, and the pain generated from, a herniated or degenerating disc. Pain relief can be felt in both the back and the leg, and when the pain is very acute the exercises may be done several times a day. The overall goal of this comprehensive exercise programme is to reduce pain, develop the muscular support of the trunk and spine, and to diminish stress to the intervertebral disc and other parts of the spine.

Of the handful of studies comparing the different exercises, McKenzie extension exercises appeared more beneficial in terms of reducing pain and stiffness than other types of exercises.

The McKenzie method not only influences mechanical changes through repeated movement and postural correction, but also encourages people to take a more active role in managing their problem.

It is helpful to have the exercises taught to you, so that they are properly explained in a useful sequence, which builds towards full pain relief and prevention of further problems. All seven exercises can, however, be undertaken at home in just five minutes a day. If you experience pain or do not notice any effect after a few days, see a McKenzie practitioner.

The McKenzie extension

This is the same type of exercise developed by McKenzie to allow the discs of the spine to shift away from the nerve roots.

While lying on your stomach, push up your chest only with both hands simultaneously while keeping your pelvis flat against the floor. Push your back up until you reach a comfortable stretch in the extended position. Do eight to twelve repetitions while holding each one for eight to ten seconds at a time. You should feel no pain with this exercise, only a pulling up of the spine as the back goes into extension.

Lying face-down pain relief

This is used in the treatment of acute back pain that tends to be short-lived.

Lay face-down with your arms beside your body and your head turned to one side. Stay in this position, take a few deep breaths and then relax completely for four to five minutes. Make a conscious effort to remove all tension from the muscles in your lower back.

Lying face-down in extension

Lie with your face down. Place your elbows under your shoulders so that you lean on your forearms. Take in a few deep breaths and allow the muscles in your lower back to relax completely. Stay in this position for about five minutes.

Extension in standing position

Stand upright with your feet slightly apart. Place your hands in the small of your back with your fingers pointing backwards and your thumbs pointing forwards. Bend your trunk backwards at the waist as far as you can, using your hands as a support on which to pivot. It is important that you keep your knees straight as you do this. Once you have maintained this position for a second or two, you should return to the starting position. Each time you repeat this movement cycle, you should try to bend a little further.

This movement works to decrease the strain on your back.

Once you have fully recovered and no longer have lower back pain, this exercise is your main tool to prevent further back problems.

Hip flexor stretch

This will help to stretch and flex the lower back, upper thigh and hip area.

Lie on your back near the edge of your bed, holding your knees to your chest. Slowly lower one leg down, keeping your knee bent,

The hip flexor stretch will help to flex and stretch the lower back.

until a stretch is felt across top of your hip and thigh. Hold for 20 seconds, then relax. Repeat five times on each side.

Piriformis stretch

'Piriformis syndrome' is caused by the piriformis muscle irritating the sciatic nerve, which is experienced as pain in the buttocks, and pain from the back of your thigh to the base of the spine.

The Piriformis stretch helps with the pain of sciatica.

Lie on your back, left hip and knee flexed. Grasp your left knee with your right hand and pull the knee towards your right shoulder. In this position, grasp just above your left ankle with your left hand, and rotate the ankle outwards. Hold for 20 seconds and then relax. Repeat five times on each side.

Psoas major stretch

Psoas major is a muscle that runs down one side of your spinal column in your lower back; if it is tight, your mobility can be very limited. This muscle often causes back pain that makes it difficult to kneel or stand for extended periods.

Kneel on your right knee, your left foot flat on the floor and your left knee bent. Rotate your right leg outward. Place your hand on the muscle in your right buttock and tighten it. Lean forward through your hip, careful not to bend your lower spine. You should feel the stretch in the front of your right hip. Hold for about 30 seconds and then repeat with your left leg.

Working with a Swiss ball

Exercise balls (so-called 'Swiss balls' because they were first used in the 1960s in Switzerland to help children with cerebral palsy) have been around for some time, but are gaining in popularity with health practitioners due to the many benefits derived from their use. Simply sitting on the ball requires use of postural muscles, so using them in place of a chair when working at the computer or reading can help to strengthen the spine and improve posture, thereby reducing pain.

Bouncing up and down on the ball will help increase the stability of the spine by helping to coordinate your muscles. Studies show that this type of exercise (called 'proprioceptive input') can help reduce the likelihood of injuring an area. For information on purchasing a Swiss ball, *see* p. 104. The exercise ball can be used for a variety of purposes, including:

✔ learning a 'neutral spine' position;
✔ developing correct posture;
✔ increasing the mobility of your lower back;
✔ improving the strength of your abdomen and back muscles;

✔ developing control and strength in your 'core' body muscles;

✔ increasing your stability and balance.

Some experts suggest that you just sit on the ball for 30 minutes a day and bounce lightly, continually finding and maintaining your balance. Or try the exercises below, which can be undertaken in just five minutes a day. A Swiss ball can be purchased from a wide number of websites and many NHS physiotherapists provide them onsite and for home use.

Lumbar stabilisation exercises with Swiss ball
Make sure that you keep your abdominal muscles contracted throughout (*see* Wall squats on p. 106). The further the ball is from your body, the harder the exercise. Perform each of the exercises for 60 seconds.

Lie on your back with your knees bent and your calves resting on ball. Then:

a. Slowly raise your arm over your head and then lower your arm, alternating right and left sides.
b. Slowly straighten one knee and relax, alternating right and left sides.
c. Slowly straighten one knee and raise the opposite arm over your head. Alternate opposite arms and legs.
d. Slowly 'walk' ball forward and backward with your legs.

Sitting exercise with Swiss ball
Again, keep your abdominal muscles contracted, and

do each exercise for 60 seconds. Sit on the ball with your hips and knees bent at 90 degrees and your feet resting on the floor.

a. Slowly raise your arm over your head and then lower your arm, alternating right and left sides.

b. Slowly raise and lower your heel, alternating right and left sides.

c. Slowly raise one heel and the opposite arm over your head. Alternate opposite arm and heel.

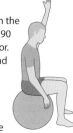

Sitting with a Swiss ball.

d. Slowly raise one foot 5 cm (2 in) from the floor, alternating right and left sides, as though you are marching.

Wall and Swiss ball

Stand with the ball between your lower back and the wall. Slowly bend your knees to 45 to 90 degrees. Hold for five seconds. Straighten your knees. Next, bend your knees to 45 to 90 degrees while raising both arms over your head.

Stomach over Swiss ball

Keep your abdominals contracted and do each exercise for 60 seconds. Lie on your stomach over the ball.

a. Slowly raise alternate arms over your head.

b. Then slowly raise alternate legs 5–10 cm (2–4 in) off the floor.

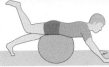

Stomach over Swiss ball. Keep your abdominal muscles firm when you do this exercise.

c. Combine exercises a and b, alternating opposite arms and legs.

d. Bend one knee. Slowly lift this leg up, alternating right and left legs. Be careful not to arch your lower back.

Heel raises

This stretching exercise improves flexibility, and releases tense muscles that might be contributing to lower back pain.

Stand with your weight spread evenly on both feet. Slowly raise your heels up and down. Repeat ten times.

Wall squats

Stand with your back leaning against the wall. Walk your feet 30 cm (12 in) in front of your body. Keep your abdominal muscles tight while slowly bending both knees to 45 degrees. Hold for five seconds. Slowly return to the upright position. Repeat ten times.

Heel raises release tense muscles and improve flexibility (*above*). Wall squats work to strengthen your back, hips and legs (*right*).

BACK RELIEF THROUGH STRETCH

The benefits of exercise for back pain are now well established; however, what isn't so clear is the fact that stretching can be one of the most important elements of any exercise programme. And here's why: stretching can help to reduce pain by loosening tension, cramps and tightened muscles, and even trapped nerves. It helps to keep muscles and ligaments flexible, as well as reducing stress on the joints. Regular stretching also improves your circulation, so that blood, oxygen and nutrients reach all parts of your back, preventing stiffness and increasing mobility and the overall health of your back.

It's important that stretching is a gentle, fluid action, with no jerking or twisting. Some people find it helps to envision a strong, flexible, healthy back and body while they stretch. Stretching exercises can be done several times a day for just a few moments, and can be incorporated easily into daily life. For example, in Chapter 2 (p. 69) there is a morning stretch to help you ease stiffness before getting out of bed. Pilates offers a wonderful stretching programme which, once learned, can be easily implemented.

As always, before undertaking exercises of any kind it's important to check with your doctor. Ensure that you feel warm and comfortable while exercising and stop if there is any sensation of pain. One of the huge benefits of stretching is that it warms the muscles – in advance of other exercise, or indeed any activity. Beginning and ending your day with stretching, and stretching whenever you feel cold, stiff or painful, can make a big difference to the health of your back and your pain.

Good breathing is also important. Try not to hold your breath. Inhale deeply before each stretch, and exhale as you stretch. This ensures a good level of oxygenated blood in your body and prevents tension as a result of breath-holding. Whatever you do, avoid bouncing when stretching, as this forces muscles beyond appropriate limits. Hold your stretches for 10 or 20 seconds, and then gently release.

Pilates

Pilates is an exercise technique invented for injured dancers nearly a century ago by ex-carpenter and gymnast Joseph Pilates. Pilates works in a completely different way to circuit training, gym workouts or weight machines. Their effect is to increase the bulk of the strongest muscles in the body, shortening and tightening them in the process.

Pilates does the opposite: muscles are lengthened and strengthened down to the deepest core, while making sure that the body is correctly balanced and aligned. A properly aligned body is at less risk of injury and is stronger, healthier and more flexible. Tension is reduced, as are problems with trapped or compressed nerves and other structures.

Like dance, yoga and martial arts, learning Pilates is a long-term, evolutionary process, and it is advised that you take classes – either in a group or one-to-one with a teacher. This helps to ensure that you are achieving the right alignment while undertaking the exercises, to ensure the best results. It is, however, possible to practise the exercises in just a few minutes a day at home, and to learn a few without the help of a teacher in order to achieve the benefits. You can expect:

✔ an increased and better balance between strength and flexibility;

✔ improved coordination;

✔ reduced stress and tension and improved posture;

✔ longer, stronger, more flexible muscles.

Pilates basics

Concentration It's important that you focus your thoughts on the area you are working at all times, to remain aware of how your muscles respond.

Control Once you learn to control your muscles, you can perform the movements fluidly throughout the range in which each muscle is capable of moving.

Core stability Many Pilates exercises are dedicated to strengthening the torso and building a strong core that will support the rest of the body. Core stability is referred to in almost all exercises, because it is fundamental for aligning and balancing the body, while protecting the spine.

Breathing You are encouraged to take a full breath in and then expel it completely while exercising, to ensure you gain maximum benefit from each exercise.

Precision It is absolutely crucial that you perform every step of every exercise as advised. Just a tiny movement out of place and the exercise will be less effective.

Core stability

The muscle groups around the centre of the body – in the abdomen, hips, buttocks, pelvic floor and inner thighs – all work together to keep the spine and pelvis aligned, thus promoting core stability. They are effectively a 'girdle of strength', holding all the bones, joints and abdominal organs in place. You will start to build your core stability from the moment you begin a Pilates exercise.

Core stabilisation exercises are easy to do, once you learn a few basic techniques. You can do them almost anywhere, several times each day, to start increasing your core stability.

Neutral spine

Neutral spine is the name for posture that maintains the three normal curves in your spine: one in your neck, one in your upper back, and one in your lower back. These three curves help absorb stress and impact on your body, both while you are sitting or standing still and when you move. It may seem more relaxing to let yourself slump down, but when you lose the normal curves of a neutral spine, you actually put more stress on your body. Your spine should be in the neutral position when you do core stabilisation exercises. To find your neutral spine:

Stand normally in front of a mirror with your hands on your hips, just below your waist. Allow your lower back to arch so your stomach juts forward and your buttocks stick out; notice how your hands rotate forward. Tighten the muscles around your stomach and buttocks so your lower back becomes very flat; notice how your hands rotate backward. Now go halfway between the forward and back positions. Keeping your pelvis in this neutral position, stand tall with your ears and shoulders lined up over your hips.

Practise finding your neutral spine in three positions: standing, sitting and lying on your back with your knees bent. Once you can find neutral spine in each position, you can maintain good posture for daily activities and for exercise.

Zip and hollow

The key to core stabilisation is learning to use the deep muscles of your trunk. There are several muscles involved, but this exercise focuses on the transverse abdominus, which wraps around the front of your body like a corset; it's the muscle you feel when you cough. You can do this exercise anywhere, in any position.

Lie relaxed on your back, your knees kept bent towards your chest. Keep your hands on part of the abdomen called the 'bikini patch' (the part of your body that a bikini bottom

Zip and hollow, whether sitting, standing or lying (as here), is used for most Pilates exercises.

would cover). Your thumbs should be touching the navel and your fingers resting about 5–6 cm (2 in) below your navel. Imagine that you are about to zip yourself into a tight pair of trousers. Hollow the area under your thumbs and fingers towards your spine. Keeping the pelvic nearly fixed, move your legs into the imaginary jeans. Ideally this will create a small movement. Imagine that the area under your fingers is being zipped together. Make sure you keep the rest of your body relaxed, and your pelvis in a neutral position.

Bridging

Lie on your back with your knees bent and your feet flat on the floor. Tighten your transverse abdominus with a zip and hollow (*see* left), then push with your feet and raise your buttocks up a few inches. Hold this position for five to ten seconds as you continue to breathe normally, then lower yourself slowly to the floor. Repeat ten times.

> Don't wear shoes when doing Pilates. You will need to feel your feet 'working', so bare feet or socks are best. There are many nerve endings on the soles of your feet that can help you to feel whether you are using them correctly, and shoes will hinder this process. If you are on a slippery surface, place a mat under your feet to hold them in position.

Basic Pilates exercises

The roll-up

This exercise strengthens the spine in the forward-bending direction. It also strengthens the abdominal muscles and restores the spine to normal alignment. Take care that you do not flex your knees or elbows. You'll need a floor mat or a rug to lie on.

Lie on your back, keeping your legs straight. Stretch your arms above your head while your shoulders rest on the floor mat. Let your back rest flat

The roll-up strengthens the spine and abdominal muscles.

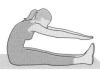

on the floor, and then slowly lift your arms straight towards the ceiling and breathe in. While breathing out, slowly roll forward with your spine peeling off the mat. Keep your head straight with your eyes looking forward. Keep your stomach taut (zipped and hollowed) and not crunched. Stretch out your legs while drawing in air through your nose. Slowly roll back on the floor. Roll up again while breathing in without a pause. Repeat these movements ten times.

Note: If you find this exercise difficult, here are a few tips/variations:

1. On the way up, place your arms under the small of your back and use your arms to help you up.

2. Bend your knees and put your feet up on a stool or a pile of cushions. They should be high enough so that when you place your legs on top of them, your knees and hips are at right angles, but your hips are firmly on the floor.

3. Hold a cushion between your knees. Keep your

knees in line with your hip joints and flex your feet very slightly.

4. Put your hands behind your head, clasping them very lightly and breathe in.

5. As you breathe out, pull your navel to the floor and then curl forward. At the top of the curl, breathe in, then uncurl again while breathing out. Make sure your abdominals are doing the work and that you are not pressing down on your heels.

The arrow

This exercise works the back extensor muscles without over-extending – and these help to stabilise your torso. This is a good one to follow a roll-up, as it balances the muscles being worked.

Lie on your stomach with a pillow under your abdomen. Rest your forehead on a paperback book or a folded towel. Your arms should be by your sides, with the palms facing upwards, and your legs should be hip-width apart and slightly rotated outwards so that your heels point in. Breathe in. Breathe out, engage your abdominals in a 'zip and hollow' movement, and let your palms float up until they are roughly level with your hips. Gently pull your shoulder blades towards your buttocks and lift your head and breastbone away from the floor without bending your head back. As you lift, you should feel the muscles below your shoulder blades working. Breathe in to return to the start. Repeat ten times.

Ballerina arms

This exercise helps to elongate your spine and improve your posture and flexibility.

1. Sit on a mat with your legs crossed. Imagine a wall behind your back and straighten your spine as if you were resting against it.

2. Protect your shoulders in their sockets by bending your elbows at a 90-degree angle. Now take your arms back in order to connect your shoulder blades.

3. Move your arms down so that the shoulder blades slide slightly down your spine.

4. Bring your arms to front and gently raise your bent arms above your head similar to the way a ballerina would.

5. Finish the exercise by moving your arms to the starting position in front of you. Repeat three or four times.

The Ballerina arms stretch helps to lengthen your spine.

The cat

This exercise stretches the whole length of the spine and is particularly good for pregnant women and anyone with lower back pain. Make sure your repetitions are smooth and flowing, with no pause in between.

Kneel on all fours with your hands shoulder-width apart and your knees hip-width apart. Hold your head so that the spine is naturally straight and your lower back is slightly curved. Breathe in and slowly round your back upwards while letting your head drop down so you are looking at your knees. You should feel the stretch right through the length of your back. Keep the movement smooth and flowing. Breathe out and engage your abdominals, then scoop your back down into a curve so that your head and bottom lift upwards. Breathe in to return to the starting point. Repeat ten times.

The saw

This is a good spine stretch, encouraging healthy spinal rotation.

Sit with your legs slightly wider than hip width, feet flexed. Your arms should be extended straight out to the sides. Sit up very straight as if you are trying to touch the ceiling with the top of your head. Exhale and turn your upper body to the left, keeping your arms in line with your shoulders, and bend as if your left hand were going to saw off your left little toe. Inhale, return slowly to your original position, and repeat to the right. Repeat ten times.

There are hundreds more Pilates exercises that are appropriate for back-pain sufferers, and all will enable you to work towards developing a strong, healthy back and good posture. Your flexibility and mobility will also be improved dramatically, and the elongation of your muscles will actually make you look and feel taller. For more details on books and other resources on Pilates, *see* p. 107.

Other stretching exercises

The following stretches are useful for anyone with back pain, loosening and lengthening. Do each of them three to five times, whenever you get a chance. In just five minutes a day, you will notice a difference in your flexibility.

Neck stretches

Stand with your feet flat on the floor, knees slightly bent, head forward. Tilt your head slowly forward, bringing your chin towards your chest. Turn your head to the left very slowly until your chin is aligned with your left shoulder. Repeat to the right. Tilt your head slowly to the left, bringing your ear over your left shoulder. Repeat to the right. Return to the starting position.

Hamstring stretch

Lay flat on your back with your knees bent. Grasp one leg behind the thigh and slowly bring it towards your chest. Pull until a gentle stretch is felt. Hold. Return to starting position. Alternate legs.

Hip twists

Lay flat on your back with your knees bent. Keeping your back flat on the floor, slowly rotate your hips to the left, lowering your legs down to the floor until you feel a mild stretch. Hold. Return to the starting position. Repeat, rotating your hips to the right. Hold. Return to the starting position.

Back extensions

Lie on your stomach. Prop yourself up on your elbows, extending your back. Slowly straighten your elbows, further extending your back, until you feel a mild stretch. Hold. Return to the starting position. Take your time.

Increasing your flexibility and mobility can take some time, particularly if your back is very painful or you have suffered from back problems for some time. You may find some of the exercises difficult at the outset, but take it slowly and perform only as many repetitions as you feel comfortable with, stopping if you feel any pain whatsoever. A gentle pulling or loosening sensation is what you are aiming for. Over a few weeks, the effects will become obvious.

BACK RELIEF THROUGH YOGA

Yoga has long been considered an important discipline for back-pain sufferers, and there are a number of key benefits. Yoga helps to increase strength in muscles and muscle groups by teaching you holding positions and incorporating gentle movements. Many yoga postures gently strengthen the muscles in the back and the abdomen, which help you to maintain a proper upright posture and movement. When these muscles are strong and flexible, back pain can be greatly reduced or avoided.

Yoga incorporates stretching and relaxation, which reduces tension in stress-carrying muscles. For people with lower back pain, stretching is very important. For example, stretching the hamstring muscles (in the back of the thigh) helps to expand the motion in the pelvis, decreasing tension across the lower back. As with other stretching disciplines, yoga improves circulation, encouraging the flow of blood, oxygen and nutrients to the muscles and soft tissues in the lower back.

Yoga poses are designed to train the body to be healthy and supple. Consistent practice and application will result in improved posture and an increased sense of balance, with your head, shoulders and pelvis in proper alignment. Proper body alignment and good posture, which helps maintain the natural curvature of the spine, are important parts of reducing or avoiding lower back pain.

Yoga breathing exercises (*pranayama*) gently work the muscles of the upper back. The yoga breathing exercises and postures also have the potential to reduce much of the tension and stress that can contribute to back pain. A primary focus of yoga is therapeutic relaxation through gentle exercise and meditation. Yoga teachers believe that by focusing the mind inwards you will be able to relax profoundly, revitalise your body and achieve a greater sense of harmony and well-being. Yoga can help you to be aware of your body and emotions and can alert you to what it is that actually brings on your back pain.

Caution

Be sure to get advice from a trained teacher before beginning any yoga programme. There are a vast number of positions (*asanas*) that will be hugely beneficial for back pain. But there are some that can exacerbate it, or which need to be adjusted to take into consideration the cause of your problems.

Pranayama – yoga breathing

Yoga breathing, or *pranayama*, is the science of breath control. It consists of a series of exercises especially intended to meet the body's needs and keep it in vibrant health. The word *pranayama* means 'breathing techniques' or 'breath control'. Ideally, this practice of opening up the inner life force is not merely to take healthy, deep breaths. It is intended for yoga practitioners to prepare and assist them in their meditation process.

Ideally, *pranayama* exercises should be carried out while you are lying on your back or sitting down, although they can be done anywhere. Make sure you keep your head and back in alignment. Practise the exercises for five minutes every morning and evening.

As you practise, count slowly to yourself until you have mastered the art of breathing in a relaxed way.

Vitality breath

Take a deep breath in through both nostrils. To exhale, pull in your abdominal muscles and diaphragm in a sharp stroke that forces the air out of your nose so quickly that the breath is almost a sneeze. As soon as you have exhaled, relax, then allow the breath to be inhaled naturally in a short burst. Exhalation should take less time than inhalation. To begin with, perform the vitality breath ten times at a rate of two exhalations per second. This completes one cycle. Take a minute's rest between ending one cycle and beginning the next. Begin by completing two cycles and gradually build yourself up to five.

Complete breath

Breathe in deeply from your abdomen, which will expand from the rib cage and up to your collarbone. Breathe out, feeling yourself deflate in a reversal of the inhalation. Give your abdomen a gentle push to help clear the breath from the bottom of your lungs. Breathe in deeply to a slow count of four, then out, again to a count of four. As you become more practiced at the exercise, gradually increase to the count of eight.

Alternate nostril breathing

Alternate nostril breathing is considered the most important of all *pranayamas* because it helps to purify and energise the system. Assume a comfortable sitting position, and rest your left hand on your left knee. Take a few breaths. Shut your right nostril with your right thumb. Exhale slowly through your left nostril. Inhale slowly and deeply through your left nostril, keeping your right nostril closed. Then, take your thumb from your right nostril and close your left nostril with the little finger and ring finger of your right hand. Exhale through your right nostril. Without stopping, inhale through your right nostril, keeping your left nostril closed. Then close your right nostril and exhale through your left. This comprises one round of alternate nostril breathing. Repeat the process a few times. Inhalation and exhalation should be done very slowly and soundlessly.

Yoga for back pain

The following exercises or positions are particularly good for back pain. Move into the poses slowly and gently; use long hold times and practise slow, deep breathing in the poses.

Any movements that increase your symptoms should be avoided. If a yoga pose causes any pain, tingling or numbness, stop immediately. All movements should be gentle, and held for the suggested period of time.

The cat

This exercise helps to open up space in the spinal column and helps to release tightness or tension from the back of the body. Put yourself in an all-fours position, with hands and knees on the floor. Your calves and feet should be relaxed, with 90-degree angles at the knees, hips and shoulders. Inhale and drop your abdomen towards the floor, looking up. Exhale while pushing into your hands, taking your spine to the sky and dropping your head to look towards your abdomen. Hold each position for five to ten seconds.

The cobra

Lay face-down with your feet together and your toes pointing behind you. Place your hands flat on the floor close to your body and beside your ribcage.

As you inhale, gently push off your hands, lifting your head and chest off the ground and tilting your head back. Feel your chest moving forward as well as upward; this will help you keep from straining the lower back. Don't be surprised if you can't raise your chest very far. This pose usually involves a small, subtle motion, at least at first.

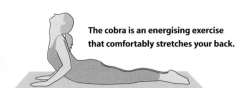

The cobra is an energising exercise that comfortably stretches your back.

The plough

Lie down with your back on a mat. Your shoulders should lie on the edge and your head should on the mat. Your legs should be straight and pressed together gently at the knees. Lift your legs off the floor with your hips following, raising your legs up, over and beyond your head. Lift your back and move your legs further beyond your head. Straighten your spine and keep your back straight. Move your hands towards your back. Place your arms against your upper back and try to move your hands as near as possible to your shoulder blades. Try to place your

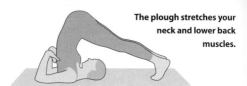

The plough stretches your neck and lower back muscles.

elbows at shoulder width. If you cannot do this, put them at a somewhat wider distance from each other. Try to relax the shoulders and the neck muscles through your breathing. Slowly bring your legs, one by one, back to the mat, stretch your arms lengthwise away from you and slowly roll your back downwards, vertebra by vertebra.

Warning: Do not try this pose if you are currently experiencing back pain.

Knee to chest

This pose encourages circulation to your back muscles and helps to relieve tension and tightening.

Lie flat on your back, with your body relaxed. Slowly and deliberately, bring one knee up towards your chest. Place your hands underneath your knee (on the back of your leg) and gently pull towards your chest. Hold for 10 to 15 seconds, feeling the stretch in the hamstring, before slowly lowering the knee back down. Repeat with your other leg.

Seated spinal twist

This pose opens your chest, relaxes tight shoulders, realigns your spine and tones your abdomen, all of which will help with back pain.

Sit down and straighten your legs out in front. Bend your left knee towards your chest and bring the heel of your left foot close to your left hip. Hook your left arm around your left knee, with your palm facing upwards and outwards. Inhale and twist to the right, turning your head away from your upright knee. Bring your right arm slowly down and behind your back until it meets (or almost meets) your left hand. It should look as though you have brought a classic ballerina arm pose downwards at the back. Breathe gently. Turn your head and body as far as you can away from the upright knee and hold. Keep your spine, neck and head aligned and continue to try to turn to the right. Breathe in and out for 60 seconds and repeat to the other side.

Seated spinal twist works on many parts of your body to open and realign.

Palm tree

The pose fully stretches the upper part of the body, encouraging flexibility. It also expands the ribcage and strengthens the muscles of the neck, lower back, abdomen and pelvis. This *asana* can be done anywhere, and within a short period of time, making it very versatile.

Stand erect. Keep your feet slightly turned out and sufficiently apart according to your height and build. Look straight ahead. Inhaling, slowly raise your arms overhead with the palms facing each other. Raise your heels slowly, keeping your balance. Lift yourself onto your toes slowly until you stand on tiptoe. Exhale slowly and keep balance. Inhale slowly again. Balancing the body on tiptoe, pull up and stretch your arms upwards from the shoulder blades with the fingers outstretched. Raise your heels as high as possible and stretch your body to the maximum. Stretch your neck and head backwards and look up. Hold your breath and keep your balance.

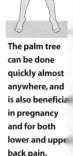

The palm tree can be done quickly almost anywhere, and is also beneficia in pregnancy and for both lower and uppe back pain.

Keep yourself firmly in this position for as long as you can hold your breath comfortably. Exhaling, relax the body and return to the starting position by slowly lowering your arms and heels simultaneously, bending your neck and head forwards.

Seated forward bend

This is an excellent stretch for the whole of the back of your body, and it is known to be very calming.

Sit down with your legs stretched. Your legs should be together, with your toes pointing upwards.

Look forwards, lengthen your back, and keep your chest and breathing free. Slowly bend forwards from the hips, stretching your crown upwards. Avoid moving or tilting your legs. When you can't bend any further, move your hands to your lower legs, ankles or feet. Lightly pull your legs, ankles or feet and continue stretching. Keep your shoulders down. Breathe in and out deeply and in a relaxed way across the entire length of your spinal column . Every time you exhale, you should bend further towards your legs without losing the length in your back. Gently release your grip and let your forearms fall to the floor, palms relaxed and facing upwards or slightly inwards. Now stretch your arms forwards. Slowly raise your upper body. Keep your legs together and toes pointing upwards. Sit up straight again, breathing regularly.

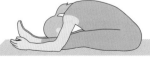

Seated forward bend. This posture can be useful in pregnancy.

BACK RELIEF THROUGH WALKING

There are several reasons why walking will help ease your back pain, not only because it is an excellent low-impact form of aerobics, which has been shown to reduce the incidence of back pain, but also because it works to strengthen muscles in the legs, hips and torso, and increases the stability of the spine. Walking also improves circulation, which encourages oxygen, blood and nutrients into the soft tissues of your body. It improves flexibility and encourages a greater range of motion, which can protect against future injuries. What's more, because it is a weight-bearing exercise, it helps to strengthen your bones and prevent osteoporosis.

Walking is ideal because it can be done almost anywhere, with few, if any, props. Good shoes are important, and many walkers wish to invest in a pedometer, to keep track of the number of steps they walk. Little else is required.

Starting a programme

It's extremely important that you do some gentle stretching to warm your muscles before walking. This increases the range of motion and helps to prevent cramps and tension in your muscles.

Try to walk quickly, but take care that you can still maintain a conversation (so you are not, effectively, too breathless). If it becomes painful at any time, slow down, or stop and stretch for a few minutes.

There are several ways to work out a programme that is right for you. First of all, you could aim for 10,000 steps a day. If you are quite unfit, or haven't been active for some time, begin with 3,000 and try to add 200 steps every other day until you reach the 10,000-step target.

Alternatively, begin with a five-minute daily walk, and go for a few minutes longer on each outing, until you can walk quickly and comfortably for 20 or 30 minutes, ideally three or four times every week.

Learn good walking form. This is very important because it ensures good posture and optimises the use of your muscles and other structures. Try to utilise the Alexander Technique head-neck balance,

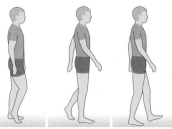

Make sure you utilise the head-neck balance while walking. Hold your arms in this position for a gentle walk, but put them up at 90-degree angles when walking quickly.

maintaining the length and width of your spine while walking (*see* p. 49). Your head should be upwards and forwards, with your eyes focused ahead. Keep your shoulders relaxed, but straight.

To maintain good posture, stretch your spine tall, reaching up to the sky with the top of your head. Your head should be resting in line with your spine. Don't tilt it back or tuck your chin in. This is especially important when walking up hills, as looking up the hill can strain your neck and make it harder to breathe.

With your spine tall, contract your stomach muscles slightly and lift them upwards to support your lower back. This will help to maintain a good posture as well as avoiding straining your lower back.

When walking up hill it is natural to lean into the hill; however, try and keep this to a minimum, maintaining an upright posture instead. Incorrect posture can lead to considerable back pain and imbalance.

Keep your body upright as you walk downhill. This may feel as if you are leaning backwards opposite the slope of the hill. Your pace should increase your breathing rate even to the point where you are slightly winded, however if you cannot talk and are completely out of breath you are over-exerting yourself. Allow the ground to support you, and think of a lengthening of the spine. The idea is neither to be fixed nor slumped, but with your weight centred so you are not leaning forwards or backwards from the hip joints.

Your strides should feel natural; don't make the mistake of thinking that long strides are more effective. You should feel comfortable – and comfortably upright. Keep your arms close to your body. Ideally, they should be at a relaxed angle, and should keep in motion, swinging from front to back, in pace with the stride of the opposite leg. Keep your hands relaxed at all times. Slower walks should be more natural, with your arms moving gently in rhythm with your strides, and hanging more freely or raised into a comfortable, relaxed position by your sides.

With each step, put your foot down firmly on your heel and midfoot, and then roll smoothly to push off with your toes.

The right shoes

Good walking shoes are a crucial piece of equipment, not only because they will maximise the benefits of walking, but also to support and protect your back. The wrong shoes will throw you off balance, changing your natural posture and the alignment of your spine, leading to muscle strain and back pain. According to US chiropractor Dr Ted Forcum, Director of the Back in Motion Sports Injuries Clinic in Oregon, there are several things to look out for:

Walking shoes should allow the feet to roll naturally slightly inwards (pronation) and outwards (supination) to help absorb the different forces acting on the body. For many people, either one or both feet under-pronate (roll outwards) or over-pronate (roll inwards), altering the balance and length of the leg while standing, as well as while walking. Some shoes are designed to control over-pronation; others are designed to encourage pronation. Therefore it is important to make sure that walking shoes match each individual's specific biomechanical pattern.

So take some time to ask questions about the best shoes for the job. Otherwise, look for a shoe that:

✔ feels stable throughout a range of motion;
✔ is flexible at the base of the toes, providing smooth motion;
✔ is comfortable, with padding and contours that neatly fit your foot – snug at the heel and midfoot; but with plenty of room for your toes to move around.
✔ Consider purchasing a removable shoe insert if the arch in the shoe doesn't support your own arch, or if it feels wrong or uncomfortable.

Five-minute walks

There are three ideal times to take short walks, and even if you can fit in only one or two, you will be doing a great deal for your back. While short walks aren't enormously beneficial to your cardiovascular health, and therefore don't specifically rank as aerobic exercise, they do make a difference to your pain and level of comfort, and help you work towards your 10,000-step target per day.

Pre-breakfast walk

This helps to stretch out the stiffness and discomfort caused by the muscles being inactive during sleep. It also encourages blood flow and circulation, which may have been stagnant overnight. It warms your muscles so that your morning activities are less likely to be painful or to cause damage or injury, and lifts your mood in advance of the day.

Lunchtime walks

Many corporations now suggest lunchtime 'walking clubs' to help deal with the high number of back-related problems at work. They are a great way to loosen tense muscles, strengthen the back through regular movement, improve mobility and, once again, lift mood. Strains will benefit from an increased blood supply, and it is a good opportunity to work on your posture.

Evening walks

Many people are stiff and suffer from discomfort after a long day behind a desk or on their feet. A gentle walk helps to improve circulation, which brings blood and nutrients to the site of the pain. It helps to deal with stress by relaxing tense muscles, and warms your muscles in advance of sleep.

BACK RELIEF IN WATER

Water exercise is especially beneficial for those with back pain caused by osteoarthritis of the spine or disc problems. The buoyancy of the water supports the majority of the body weight, taking pressure off the joints and intervertebral discs. The resistant properties of water make the muscles work harder to perform movements such as walking, marching or other exercise. You can strengthen the muscles that support the back without stressing the joints and discs. The pressure the water exerts on the body prevents an injured joint from further inflammation and post-exercise back pain. Additionally, the water temperature should be warm enough to relax muscles, which also helps relieve pain.

Which exercise?

Any of the exercises in this book can be undertaken in water (doing the sitting exercises in shallow water, if possible), and the same benefits will be achieved. Walking in water up to your waist or chest is also good aerobic exercise, and even just five minutes will provide a good workout for most people.

Swimming is also excellent, but remember the following tips:

Front crawl: Do not rotate your head too far or too quickly when taking breaths. Avoid letting your head move up or down too much – keep it in line with the axis along the length of your body instead. When you aren't breathing, keep your head facing downwards. Be sure to roll your body when taking a breath and avoid jerking the head backwards so that you reduce strain on the neck.

Backstroke: The muscles along the front of your neck will become tired if you haven't done this stroke recently, so take it slowly. Make your strokes even and gentle and, if you experience any pain, stop immediately.

Breaststroke: Keep your head and neck still, while gently raising your back to take breaths. Use the momentum of your legs to raise you in the water, rather than using your neck or back.

Sidestroke: This stroke (and also the backstroke) can minimise stress on the back when compared with frontward strokes.

It is very important that you do the strokes correctly, as further injury may result from jerky, unaccomplished movements. Swimming lessons may be useful if you aren't a regular swimmer. Or, stick to water exercise until your back is feeling stronger and less painful.

Benefits of water exercise

Buoyancy: The buoyancy of water suspends the body and reverses the effects of gravity. Buoyancy offers effective partial weight-bearing support that can be enhanced by the use of flotation devices. One of the greatest benefits of water exercise is its effect on flexibility. Stretching exercises that might otherwise be difficult on land are much easier in the water, because you can move your joints through a wider range of motion and achieve long-term flexibility because the effects of gravity are lessened. In addition, water exercise acts as a cushion for weight-bearing joints.

Density: Water is denser than air, which provides increased resistance to movement. Actually, water results in more than 12 times the resistance encountered when performing the same exercises on land. It's this increased resistance in every direction that adds to the workout and is the primary reason why you can improve both strength and resistance while exercising in water. Weak lower back muscles can achieve significant strength improvement.

Hydrostatic pressure: Water also produces hydrostatic pressure to all submerged body parts. This means that the pressure from the water on the body increases with the depth of the body part. This pressure opposes the tendency of blood to pool in the lower extremities and therefore reduces any swelling.

Five-minute water exercises

Walking or jogging: In the water for five minutes.

Scissor spreads: Support yourself at the edge of the pool with both arms relaxed. If you don't know how to swim, sit on a step at the side of the pool. Spread your legs into a 'V' position and then bring them across each other, like a pair of scissors opening and closing. Alternate your right leg across your left, then left leg across right. This will require the use of abdominal muscles to maintain the position while you scissor your legs. Do this for five minutes.

Leg swings: While holding onto the edge of the pool, swing a straight leg forwards towards the surface of the water, then down and backwards. Pull backwards only within a pain-free range.

Leg circles: Standing away from the pool wall, start with very small circles. Lift your leg straight forwards, then sweep it through a smooth circular motion out to the side, then behind your body. Complete the circle by brushing your leg past your standing leg and beginning the next circle. After completing the repetitions, reverse the direction of the circle, going from clockwise to anti-clockwise.

Knee-to-chest exercise: Put one hand on the side of the pool or stand with your back to the wall. Bring your knees up to your chest gently, avoiding any jerking action. Alternating legs stretches the lower back and thigh muscles.

ALTERNATIVE METHODS

Outside the conventional medical system, there are a number of other therapeutic options that can help with your back pain. Some of these can be learned and undertaken at home; others take place in a therapist's or practitioner's office or clinic. In this chapter we'll look at some of the tried-and-tested options, and those which you can easily adapt on a DIY basis. Your GP or consultant may be in a position to refer you to some of these therapists – in particular osteopaths, chiropractors or acupuncturists – as these therapies are well established, conventionally approved in most cases, and known to have a positive effect on back pain. There is no doubt that you'll need a little more than five minutes a day for treatment to be effective, but it can be worth the time invested to go this one step further. What's more, a good practitioner will give you plenty of good advice to encourage the health of your back, and to deal with pain when it arises. One of the most important things is, of course, finding a good practitioner who you can trust, and that's where we will begin.

FINDING A PRACTITIONER

If your doctor is not in a position to refer you to a reputable practitioner, there are a number of ways to go about finding one. The first is to approach the regulatory body for the therapy you are considering. All have lists of registered and approved practitioners in your area, and many can provide you with someone who specialises in back pain. You'll find details of the regulatory bodies for each of the therapies we discuss at the back of this book (*see* pp. 188–89).

The success of alternative therapies can be enormously dependent on a good practitioner/patient relationship, and your choice of a therapist is as important as the choice of therapy. You will need to feel comfortable talking to your practitioner, and if you feel embarrassed or ill at ease you will be less likely to get across all of the essential information. A good therapist will naturally draw out the important information, and you will go away feeling reassured and comfortable.

Take your time, check the therapist's qualifications, ask for recommendations from friends, your doctor or another therapist, and do not commit yourself until you are sure you will have a rapport. Make sure that the practitioner has experience treating back pain.

While it goes without saying that all osteopaths, chiropractors and acupuncturists will have plenty of experience, other therapists may not.

The consultation

The initial consultation is the most important part of any natural therapy session. This is the first session with a therapist, and the one in which the most information is exchanged. The first session usually lasts longer than any subsequent sessions because your therapist will aim to find out all about you before any diagnosis can be made. You can expect your therapist to ask you all about:

✔ your physical condition, including past and present illnesses, any medication you are taking, any symptoms and interesting aspects to them (whether pain is sharp or dull, for example, or perhaps worse at night or in cold weather);

✔ your diet, including cravings, appetite, any weight problems, habits, obvious dislikes and reactions to foods;

✔ your sleeping patterns;

✔ home life, whether there are any obvious stresses or tension, or perhaps relationship problems or financial difficulties; similarly, you'll be asked about your work life;

✔ your exercise patterns;

✔ your emotional state;

✔ any other treatment you may be undergoing, both conventional and complementary, including any home treatments you may be doing;
✔ what you hope to get from treatment.

The most important aspect of the consultation is to get across every tiny bit of information you can summon up, no matter how trivial it may seem at the time. This presents a clear picture for the therapist, and he or she will be able to offer treatment based on all the important facts, whether they seem relevant to you or not.

Many therapists use a variety of diagnostic techniques alongside the information you provide. For example, a Traditional Chinese Medicine (TCM) practitioner will use personal touch and observation, including:

✔ pulse-taking (there is more than one pulse in TCM);
✔ hands-on examination of abdomen;
✔ posture, movement and skin-texture diagnosis;
✔ tongue diagnosis;
✔ possibly urine analysis.

Others may do a physical examination much as your doctor would, and ask to see you walk, sit and indicate how you normally hold yourself when you are working. The depth of information required differs between therapists, but don't be alarmed if you are questioned intensively; therapists don't just treat pain, they look for the root cause of it.

BACK RELIEF THROUGH OSTEOPATHY AND CHIROPRACTIC

Both chiropractors and osteopaths are trained to deal with back pain of many descriptions, including sciatica and other syndromes related to the spine. They work slightly differently in the way they approach treatment.

Chiropractic

This therapy works on the musculo-skeletal system, focusing mainly on the spine and its effects on the nervous system. The term 'musculo-skeletal' refers to the body's structures: the bones, joints, muscles, ligaments and tendons that give the body its form. Through a series of special examination and manipulative techniques, chiropractors can diagnose and treat numerous disorders associated with your back.

It is every chiropractor's aim to restore the spine to its natural, perfectly functioning state, as appropriate to each individual. Problems are diagnosed through observation and palpation (hands-on examination). X-rays are used to pinpoint the area of damage, assess the extent of the injury and decide if chiropractic treatment is suitable. Chiropractors aim to restore the spine and musculo-skeletal system to normal function by using a variety of special chiropractic manipulative techniques.

Whereas mobilisation involves moving a joint as far as it will comfortably go within its normal range of movement, manipulation involves shifting it even further with any one of a number of different techniques. Where manipulation is involved, a chiropractor will use the correct amount of force at the correct speed to thrust into the spinal joint to the correct depth. There are about 150 different techniques. Treatment may also involve soft-tissue work.

Treatment can sometimes be uncomfortable, but the type and amount of pressure used is worked out to your individual needs. Often very little force is necessary. Massage and 'trigger points' may be used to loosen knots and to warm up tense, painful muscles. Ice treatments may also be used.

Some people feel an improvement after just one treatment, but the length of time it takes for a complete recovery will depend upon your particular problem, how long you've had it and your age. It's a safe therapy, suitable for everyone, of any age, except for those who have damaged bones, or bone disease such as bone cancer. It's also appropriate for pregnancy-related back pain. Research in the UK has found chiropractic to provide 'worthwhile, long-term benefits' for patients with low back pain in comparison to hospital outpatient management. This study also found that chiropractic benefits persist for a three-year period, indicating long-term benefits.

Osteopathy

This manipulative therapy works on the body's structure (skeleton, muscles, ligaments and connective tissue) to relieve pain, improve mobility and restore all-round health. Much of osteopathic practice focuses on easing muscular tension, which does more than simply alleviate pain and stiffness. The osteopathic belief is that a relaxed muscle is a well functioning muscle – a belief based on the physiological fact that muscles use up enormous energy when they contract.

Stress, either mental or physical, can cause muscles to contract, wasting energy and making the muscles less elastic, so that they are more prone to damage. Tense muscles can also impede the flow of blood and lymph fluids, which flow through them. By relaxing tight muscles these important nutrients can flow freely, allowing blood to carry nutrients and oxygen to where they are needed, and enabling toxin and waste-carrying lymph to drain away.

Through a series of established manipulative techniques an osteopath can diagnose and treat people with all kinds of back pain (and many other physical problems, too). The techniques are chosen depending on the muscles that are being treated. Most of the techniques are not violent or usually painful. Some, however, such as a 'high-velocity thrust' are more forceful than others, but even these are not rough or painful.

An osteopath will observe you from all angles and evaluate the way your body functions before checking parts such as your spine, hips and legs. He or she will put you through a series of movements to test your joints to find out how well and with what ease you can move them; he will also palpate the tissue as it moves. Passive movement testing is also involved, which means that he will move your body and feel how it responds to the movement.

Most people need about three treatments to see any improvement, but most also respond well within five. All treatment is safe if you visit a qualified practitioner. It is not suitable for people with weak or fragile bones, such as those with severe osteoporosis; inflamed joints from rheumatoid arthritis should not be treated either, although unaffected parts of the body can be. Broken bones and those with diseases such as bone cancer are not suitable for treatment.

A 2004 study of back pain treatments, coordinated by researchers at the University of York found that spinal manipulation, in the form of chiropractic, osteopathy or manipulative physiotherapy, followed by a programme of exercise, provided significant relief of symptoms and improvement in a person's general health.

BACK RELIEF THROUGH MASSAGE

A recent study found that massage is superior to both acupuncture and self-care for back pain. Experts agree that often the best way to manage chronic back pain is to use several therapies at once, and therapeutic massage may be an important part of the package. While massage at the hands of a trained, registered massage therapist will undoubtedly provide relief from pain, there are also a number of techniques that can be undertaken at home, in just a few minutes, to ease discomfort significantly.

Massage involves manipulating the body's soft tissues with specific techniques to promote or restore health. Massage therapists use their hands to detect and treat problems in the muscles, ligaments and tendons.

There are many different types of massage, some of which work on pressure or reflex points, such as shiatsu (Japanese massage) or reflexology (see p. 179). Others concentrate on relieving specific conditions; for example, remedial massage is used to treat sports injuries and muscle strains. But basic massage techniques have been shown to promote physical and emotional healing in two ways: by a mechanical and a reflex action.

The mechanical effects of massage are the physical results of pressing, squeezing and moving the soft tissues. Depending on the techniques used, this can be relaxing or stimulating. Tense muscles can cause a sluggish circulation because they force the body's blood vessels to constrict. Massaging the muscles relaxes them and stimulates the circulation so that blood flows freely, carrying oxygen and nutrients to where they are needed.

The reflex action is an involuntary reaction of one part of the body to the stimulation of another part. Because the body, mind and emotions form one intricate organism, connected by energy channels and a complex nervous system with receptors in the skin, stimulation in one part of the body can affect several other parts. A relaxing back massage could ease leg pain – and vice versa.

A full-body massage can last 90 minutes, but it usually lasts an hour. Afterwards you may be left alone for a few minutes to 'come round'. Everyone reacts differently to massage – you may feel relaxed, energised, slightly tired or achy the next day. Your therapist may also use some essential oils, which can help encourage relaxation or stimulation – whatever is required. All oils have different qualities and effects, and when undertaking massage at home you might wish to experiment with a few (see pp. 156–7).

You can have massage therapy as often as you wish – and if your therapist thinks that it is suitable, she may suggest a course of treatment. It's particularly good for strained muscles, arthritis, sciatica and back problems, so definitely worth considering. It's effective and safe for everyone, including pregnant women, although the use of aromatherapy oils must be scrutinised if you are pregnant or on any medication. A 1990 study found that people receiving treatment reported relief from pain and muscle spasm, as well as anxiety; other benefits were improved sleep and general well-being.

Techniques

There are a variety of different strokes that can be used at home, ranging from the most delicate touch with the fingertips to focused deep-tissue work. All strokes can be varied in speed and pressure. Keeping your hands relaxed, begin working slowly and rhythmically, gradually building up speed and pressure.

As a general rule, strokes should be made firmly in the direction of the heart, and then lightly for the return stroke.

Gliding

This stroke is used a great deal in massage and is particularly useful for applying oil to the body. It can be feather-light or a firm, reassuring stroke. Keeping the fingers together and the hands outstretched, glide the hands forwards along the length of the body or limb, retaining contact with the flat of the hand. The strokes you employ can be either long or circular, using one or both hands. The function of the gliding strokes is to relax and stretch the muscles.

Kneading

Kneading is a firm stroke used on a specific area of the body to help release muscle tension and improve circulation. Gently grasp the area with both hands and make a kneading action similar to that of kneading dough.

Draining

A light to mid-pressure stroke that relaxes and stretches the muscles and improves the circulation. Use either the heel of your hand on the large areas, or your thumbs on small areas. With one hand following the other, push firmly using the heel or thumb of first one hand and then the next, travelling slowly upwards along the limb or muscles.

The draining technique relaxes and stretches muscles.

Pulling

This stroke can be used to pull and stretch the muscles of the trunk and legs. Use alternate

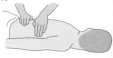

The pulling stroke stretches the muscles of the trunk and legs.

hands in a pulling motion, gradually moving them up the body.

Wringing

This stroke is similar to 'pulling' but works right across the body or limb. This is a good stroke with which to finish a particular sequence, and can be used on the torso, legs and arms. Start with your hands placed either side of the body or limb. Moving the hands in a forwards and backwards motion across the body, progress slowly towards the head.

A wringing stroke is often used to finish a particular sequence.

Friction strokes

These are deeper strokes that allow you to work around joints and into the muscles and tendons, to iron out knots and release tension. Using the thumb or fingertips, work slowly and firmly into the area, making tiny circular movements. Different individuals will prefer different pressures.

Percussive strokes

Hacking, cupping and plucking (*see below*) are used to stimulate areas, improve circulation and release muscle tension. They can be used anywhere on the body, but avoid doing them directly on the spine itself.

Hacking: With your hands open and palms facing each other, make alternating chopping motions up and down the body. As a variation on this stroke, curl the fingers into loose fists to create more of a pummelling effect on the body.

Cupping: Cup your hands and face them palms downwards. Keeping them cupped, gently beat up and down along the body.

Pinching or plucking: Gently lift small amounts of flesh or muscle and let it slide through your fingers.

Putting it into action: massaging your back

During a full-body massage the largest amount of time is usually devoted to the back and shoulders, partly because the back represents such a large part of the body and partly because this is a very common place to accumulate tension.

If you are giving someone a massage, position yourself at the person's head, and he or she should be lying on their stomach, face downwards or turned to one side, arms at their sides. Start on the upper back and glide your hands slowly down either side of the spine, back up the sides of the body and lightly over the shoulders.

Turn the person's head to the right. Work the left shoulder, using both hands, and starting at the base of the neck. Use firm strokes outwards along the shoulder and off at the top of the arm. Thumbs should be used to work into the muscles at the base

Step 1. Glide your hands slowly down either side of the spine and back up the sides of the body. Avoid rough or sudden movements.

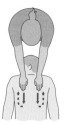

Step 2. With your partner's head turned to the left, work on the right shoulder using both hands to make firm outwards strokes.

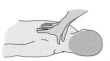

Step 3. Your thumbs should work into the muscles at the base of the neck.

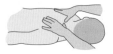

Step 4. Grasp the top of their right shoulder with your right hand and place your left hand on their lower back.

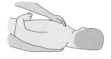

Step 5. Draw your left hand up the side of the spine, while moving your right hand down to meet your left.

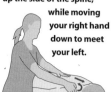

of the neck, paying particular attention to knots or areas of tightness, working firmly and slowly into the muscles, making tiny circles.

You can use a variety of different strokes on the upper back, lower back and neck and shoulder area, working the area around the shoulder blades, gliding up and down the area on either side of the spine, making kneading strokes over the hip area and gliding circles around the ribcage.

It is suggested that you massage the whole of the back, neck, legs, feet and abdomen to reduce pain and relieve tension.

Back massage in five minutes

Trigger-point release

Let the pain be your guide. What you are aiming for here is to release trigger points, using the sustained pressure of your/your partner's thumb. Ask your partner to work over any tender spots or knots that you have felt. Press firmly and gradually increase the pressure until the pain is 6 or 7 on a scale of 1 to 10. Hold the pressure until pain is reduced to about a 4. Now increase the pressure again until the pain is at 6 or 7 again, and hold until it is reduced to a 4 again. Repeat once or twice more and then apply a little warmth over the area with a hot-water bottle wrapped in a towel or a heating pad to encourage blood flow and to help maintain loose muscles.

Using oils

In many cases a masseur uses massage oil to decrease friction created on the skin and to prevent the pulling of skin. But only use a little. The less used the better, as greater friction means the pressure will be deeper. Use light stroking movements throughout a massage to move from one area to another, to soothe an area of localised tissue damage or to make a transition to another stroke. Good general oils to use as a base include:

Mineral	Almond
Soya	Grapeseed
Peach or apricot kernel	Wheatgerm
Sunflower	Aromatherapy oils

Adding 3–5 drops of different aromatherapy oils to your base oil can encourage healing, relax tense muscles, improve circulation and reduce pain. Aromatherapy oils all have their own qualities. Some of these are not appropriate for pregnancy, so please check the label before using. Those with an asterisk on the list below can also be used in a hot bath. Use the oils individually, or in a blend.

Juniper*	Pine
Lavender*	Rosemary* (will also
(will also aid sleep)	improve mood)

Ginger	Nutmeg
Thyme	Sweet marjoram*
Black pepper	Lemon (very good for
(particularly good for	swellings and
sciatic and other nerve	inflammation)
pains)	Cypress
Mandarin* (very good	Petitgrain*
for relieving stress)	Clary sage*

Ice massage

An ice massage can have an almost instant and dramatic effect on pain. Not only does it reduce inflammation and swelling, which accompanies most back pain to some degree, but it also works like an anaesthetic to numb pain. Ice slows the nerve impulses, which interrupts the pain/spasm reaction between the nerves (see p. 83); it also decreases tissue damage.

Using a block of ice, ice cubes or even frozen vegetables in a damp towel, apply the ice gently to the lower back and massage in a circular motion. Keep your movements light and local to the pain. Avoid applying the ice over the bony portion of the spine, focusing instead on the muscles around it. Work the ice over the area for five minutes (no longer). You can do this two or three times a day for almost instant relief.

BACK RELIEF THROUGH YOUR MIND

There is an increasing wealth of research indicating that your mind can have a dramatic impact on the way you perceive pain, therefore making it possible to make the pain more manageable and, in some cases, eliminating it completely.

The mind–body relationship has long been established, and we know that thoughts and emotions can directly influence physiological responses such as muscle tension, blood flow and levels of brain chemicals, which play important roles in the perception of pain.

Many back-pain sufferers notice that pain is often worse when they feel depressed or helpless; alternatively, when they are busy, happy or focused they may not find their pain as overwhelming or uncomfortable. The cause of the pain remains the same, but the way it is *perceived* is different.

There are a wide range of interventions that are aimed at working on the psychological and emotional aspects of pain. In the next section we'll look at how relaxation and meditation techniques can be used to good effect; here we'll look at some of the other options.

One 2003 study found that offering psychological support and advice helped many sufferers to overcome their back pain. Many sufferers experienced a lack of confidence, fear of movement and avoidance of certain activities, which made their lives more difficult and which prevented improvement. When encouraged or taught to deal with these factors, most of the subjects in the study experienced a return to normal activities and a considerable reduction (in some cases elimination) of pain.

Positive thinking

Another recent study found that positive thinking was as powerful as a shot of morphine for relieving pain and reducing activity in the parts of the brain that process pain information. Researchers in the US concluded that the 'brain can powerfully shape pain, and we need to exploit its power'.

One way to do this is to encourage positive thinking through affirmations. The idea is that positive affirmations change the way we think, and are a powerful tool for reprogramming our subconscious.

Positive affirmations in five minutes a day

Positive affirmations must be positive. In other words, they are statements that replace negative thought patterns and encourage the brain to think positively.

First listen carefully to your thoughts when you are in pain. 'I can't bear this,' 'I can't stand the pain,' 'I can't move,' 'This is getting worse,' 'I'll never get better,' are all common thoughts that fill our minds, and they are all negative.

Begin by replacing them with a vivid picture of their opposite; for example,

'I am feeling better every day.'

'I'm feeling more mobile.'

'I can bear this.'

'The healing has started.'

Don't use an affirmation that is unbelievable to you. It isn't going to be believable to say, for example 'I am completely pain free' if you are hurting. What you need is something positive that you can believe. Here is an example to begin with: 'I'm feeling more relaxed and comfortable' or 'My back is getting stronger and healthier every day.'

It is extremely important that your statement is couched in positive terms. If you say, for instance, 'I am not in pain,' your brain sees an image of you in pain; it doesn't interpret the 'not' word.

Write your affirmations down and repeat them for five minutes, first thing every morning or, indeed, whenever you think of it. When pain strikes, put the negative firmly out of your mind and repeat your positive affirmation statements. Write out as many as you can and repeat them over and over on an audio tape, which you can play in your car or while you are going about housework. Change the words you use for your pain. Instead of using 'indescribable', 'agony', 'debilitating' or even 'pain', choose 'ache', 'discomfort', 'sore' or 'uncomfortable'.

Remember, too, that self-limiting statements like 'I can't handle this!' or 'This is impossible!' are particularly damaging because they increase your stress in a given situation and they stop you from searching for solutions. One of the things that therapists and counsellors do when they help you to overcome the psychological or emotional aspects of your back pain is to solve problems by thinking positively about solutions. So the next time you try to get out of bed and find that your back seizes up, avoid the 'I can't do this' thinking and focus instead on 'How can I handle this?' or 'What's possible?'.

Distraction

Many people suffering from chronic pain become isolated and are left with nothing to focus on but their pain and misery. Learning to fill your mind with pleasant thoughts helps alleviate your distress. Recently, researchers have systematically evaluated several different kinds of distraction strategies for dealing with pain. A review done at the University of Pittsburgh Pain Evaluation and Treatment Institute concluded that distraction approaches can be classified into five groups. All of these have been found to be effective for mild-to-moderate pain:

pleasant images – conjure up peaceful, pain-free visions;

dramatised images – envision situations that use the pain as part of the script (for example, imagining that you are a wounded spy trying to escape your captors);

neutral images – think of your plans for the weekend;

focusing on the environment – instead of paying attention to your body, count the ceiling tiles or plan how to redecorate the room, etc.;

rhythmic activity – such as counting, reciting a poem, singing, etc.

Imagery is not a substitute for more active ways of coping with pain. But it can be a valuable part of an overall pain-management plan.

Cognitive restructuring

Our thoughts can have a profound effect on our mood and physical state, including your perception of physical pain. If you constantly tell yourself, 'I don't see how this pain is ever going to get better,' or 'I can't take it anymore,' you may exacerbate your pain in three ways:

It becomes hard to develop the sense of power and control necessary to fight the pain.

These self-defeating, stressful thoughts can further tense your muscles.

Such thoughts may alert the nervous system to widen the 'pain gate' and increase the discomfort.

Cognitive restructuring revises the way you think about your problem by rewriting your internal 'script'. In cognitive restructuring you use a diary to record: when your pain is particularly severe; what the situation was at the time of the pain; what you thought about and felt before, during and after the pain episode; and what you tried to do to decrease the pain. By examining this diary you can identify negative thoughts and feelings and learn to change them, using relaxation, positive affirmations (*see* pp. 159–61), visualisation (*see* pp. 160–62) or by getting some help from a cognitive behavioural therapist (*see* below).

Cognitive Behavioural Therapy (CBT)

A 2006 study from Holland found that people with lower back pain can reap as much benefit from CBT as they do from physical therapy. Like cognitive restructuring, CBT is a combination of cognitive therapy, which can modify or eliminate your unwanted thoughts and beliefs, and behavioural therapy, which can help you to change your behaviour in response to those thoughts.

Cognitive techniques (such as challenging negative thoughts) and behavioural techniques (such as exposure therapy that gradually desensitises you to a fear of moving or lifting, and relaxation techniques) are used to relieve symptoms by changing your thoughts, beliefs and behaviour.

CBT is based on the assumption that most unwanted thinking-patterns and emotional and behavioural reactions are learned over a long period of time. The aim is to identify the thinking that is causing your unwanted feelings and behaviours and to learn to replace this thinking with more positive thoughts.

Your therapist does not focus on the events from your past (such as your childhood) but instead focuses on current difficulties at the present time. Your therapist will be able to teach you new skills and new ways of reacting. A treatment plan is agreed, as well as a list of achievable goals, and you are likely to need somewhere in the region of eight sessions of one hour each. You have to take an active part, and are given 'homework' between sessions. The exercises can be used throughout the treatment and long after to control your pain – often in just minutes.

Although CBT with the help of a trained therapist is best, some people prefer to tackle their problems themselves. There are a range of books and leaflets on self-help for problems which CBT is useful for (anxiety, phobias, depression, etc). More recently, interactive CDs, DVDs and websites have been developed and evaluated for self-directed CBT for a variety of conditions.

BACK RELIEF THROUGH RELAXATION AND MEDITATION

Relaxation is often a part of combined medical and behavioural programmes for chronic back pain and it has, in various studies, been shown to be effective in reducing pain, muscular tension, the use of medication and depression.

True relaxation is a healing process that focuses on calming the mind and body. It involves turning your attention inward to control and resolve problems, such as stress and pain (which are often interlinked), rather than suppressing them with short-term methods such as drugs. Relaxation is an acquired skill, but once learned it can be used in five-minute bursts throughout the day to help control and even eliminate your back pain.

Relaxation works by rebalancing the sympathetic and parasympathetic parts of the autonomic nervous system. The sympathetic system deals with how the involuntary systems of the body work (such as heartbeat, circulation, breathing, etc). It is the system involved in the 'fight or flight' response which occurs when we are stressed. There is a strong connection between stress and back pain (see p. 39). Anxiety causes a release of stress hormones, which increase the perception of pain and also causes muscle tension, which can lead to painful spasm.

Relaxation frees the mind from stress and pain, allowing the muscles to relax, and switches the way the brain and nervous system work into a state where rest and repair can take place.

Therapists use and teach different techniques to bring about physical and mental relaxation, and many of these can be used quickly and successfully at home.

There are many relaxation techniques, from simple deep-breathing exercises (see p. 170), which are easy to learn on your own, to self-hypnosis and hypnotherapy (see box, pp. 168–9). The following exercises may take a little time to learn, but can be done easily in five or ten minutes each day to relieve tension and put your body into a state of healthy relaxation.

Progressive muscle relaxation

Lie on your back in a comfortable position. Allow your arms to rest at your sides, palms down, on the surface next to you. Inhale and exhale slowly and deeply. Clench your hands into fists and hold them tightly for 15 seconds. As you do this, relax the rest of your body. Visualise your fists contracting, becoming tighter and tighter. Then let your hands relax. On relaxing, visualise a golden light flowing into your entire body, making all your muscles soft and pliable. This is called 'creative visualisation', which uses the power of your mind to enhance relaxation by giving it positive images to accept.

Now, tense and relax the following parts of your body in this order: face, shoulders, back, stomach, pelvis, legs, feet and toes. Hold each part tensed for 15 seconds and then relax your body for 15 seconds before going on to the next part.

Finish the exercise by shaking your hands and imagining the remaining tension flowing out of your fingertips.

Autogenic relaxation

If tensing your muscles in the progressive muscle relaxation technique aggravates your pain, you may prefer this relaxation technique. It is called autogenic relaxation. Lie down, or sit in a comfortable chair that supports your head. Concentrate on the following muscle groups:

✔ hands and arms;
✔ feet, calves, thighs, buttocks;
✔ chest, abdomen, lumbar (lower back) region;
✔ shoulders, neck, head and face.

Begin to breathe deeply but naturally, allowing tension to ease with each exhalation. Begin by saying to yourself: 'My right hand is heavy; my right hand is relaxed and heavy and warm; my right hand is completely limp and relaxed.'

Repeat the phrases and feel the relaxation

happening. Take some time repeating the phrases three or four times before moving on to your left hand and arm. You may wish to practise this for a few days before going on to the next muscle group.

When you feel ready to move to the second group of muscles, repeat the phrases, concentrating on each of the three further muscle groups in turn. Don't rush it, relax into it without any force of will. Just let it happen. Allow your mind to be still without effort.

Hypnosis

Whether you choose to self-hypnotise or visit a hypnotherapist for your back pain, you can expect some good results. According to current research, the ability of hypnosis to increase pain tolerance and decrease pain sensation makes it effective for the treatment of chronic musculo-skeletal pain. In one study patients reported a reduction in chronic pain, increased psychological well-being and improved sleep quality. In another study comparing hypnosis to relaxation in the management of chronic low-back pain, both groups showed significant reductions in the average level of pain, the level of depression, and the length of pain. Hypnosis was more effective than a standard relaxation technique in reducing the time it took to fall asleep and in physicians' rating of patients' use of medication (the latter being less problematic after treatment).

Hypnotherapy could be described as a form of psychotherapy that works on the subconscious to change thought and behavioural patterns. The word 'hypnosis' refers to a trance-like state somewhere between waking and sleeping, which you enter when you are hypnotised; 'hypnotherapy' is the practice of bringing about healing or facilitating change while under hypnosis. A hypnotherapist uses simple techniques to induce a light trance, in which you are more suggestible and compliant. Suggestions are made which are stored in your mind, effectively reprogramming it. For example, although pain may be a physical sensation, it is one that registers in the brain. If, under hypnosis, your mind accepts that you do not feel pain, then you will not feel it.

The mechanism for pain relief is not clear, but a recent study found that when hypnotised patients were scanned, the activity in the pain centres of the brain was markedly less than that in other areas, which suggests that hypnosis does alter the way our brains perceive pain.

For details of contacting a registered hypnotherapist, *see* Further Resources (p. 189); self-hypnosis can be learned from a good therapist, or through CDs and other interactive resources.

Meditation

Meditation is known to bring about a healthy state of relaxation by decreasing the response of the sympathetic nervous system and thus reducing heart rate, respiration rate, etc.

There are two basic approaches to meditation, both of which serve to calm the mind: focusing the attention on a specific object or concept (concentration meditation, *see* below); keeping moment-to-moment awareness of the flow of experience by *observing* rather than *reacting* to it.

Several studies have investigated the effect of meditation on chronic pain from a variety of causes. Positive results include a higher pain tolerance, decreased anxiety and depression, increased activity levels, decreased use of pain-related medications, and increased levels of self-esteem.

Easy concentration meditations

Objects of meditation can include your breathing, an image you visualise in your mind or a real image you look at, such as a candle flame or sacred icon. One purpose of concentration meditation is to help you focus your attention and concentrate.

Breathe deeply If you're a beginner, consider starting with this technique. Breathing is a natural function that you won't have to consciously learn. You simply pay attention to your breathing – how it feels when air enters or leaves your nostrils. Don't follow it down to your lungs. When you feel your attention wander, gently return your focus to your breathing.

Scan your body When using this technique, you'll focus your attention on sensations such as pain, tension, warmth or relaxation in different parts of your body. Combine body scanning with breathing exercises and imagine breathing heat or relaxation into and out of different parts of your body.

Repeat a name, word or phrase A mantra is the name of a sacred deity or phrase that you repeat silently or aloud. You can create your own mantra, if you'd like. One word will do. For example, 'peace', 'relax' or 'calm'. If you are religious, you may choose to say 'Allah' or 'Jesus', for example. Block out all other thoughts, feelings and sensations. If you feel your attention wandering, bring it back to your breathing. Use the words as a sort of 'chant'; for example, as you inhale, say the word 'peace' to yourself, and as you exhale, say the word 'calm.' Draw out the pronunciation of the word so that it lasts for the entire breath. Continue this exercise until you feel very relaxed.

Many ancient exercise practices, such as yoga, Qi Gong and t'ai chi, incorporate a type of 'moving meditation' as part of the movements or postures. This type of meditation may be particularly helpful if you find it hard to sit still.

BACK RELIEF THROUGH QI GONG

This ancient Chinese system of exercises combines movement and mindfulness – a form of meditation that includes focusing on breathing and body awareness – to relax the muscles and ease stresses on the body. In 1996, the prestigious Maryland School of Medicine in the US incorporated Qi Gong into a programme for managing chronic lower back pain.

Traditional Chinese medicine practitioners believe that our vital energy (or qi) flows smoothly as long as dynamic equilibrium is maintained in energy meridians. Neck and back pain, as well as gastrointestinal and emotional pain, are understood to be areas of stagnation or interruptions in the smooth flow of qi. For Traditional Chinese Medicine practitioners, pain can evolve into more serious chronic conditions or diseases such as headaches, migraines, inability to work or function and even cancer.

It is the goal of every Qi Gong exercise to enhance the free flow of qi. Modern research shows Qi Gong exercises can address many areas of pain. There are a number of different postures and series of postures. It's a good idea to begin by taking a Qi Gong class, where an instructor will take you through the movements and encourage you to focus and breathe correctly. Movements are often very small – even imperceptible – but they work on key areas of the body that will release your vital energy or qi.

Qi Gong in five minutes a day

Exercise 1. Arm swings

Begin with your feet firmly planted shoulder-width apart. Rotate on your heels while turning left to right from your hips. Your arms will hang limply at your sides, swinging as your lower body turns from side to side. Lead from your hips, not from your shoulders. Breathe consciously, in and out through your nose, with deep, slow breaths from your diaphragm. Practise for five minutes in the morning or evening (or both) to prevent stagnation and pain in your back, hips, knees and shoulders.

Exercise 2.
Turning like a windmill in a calm breeze

This exercise will help to encourage the flow of qi, and the mild bends and rotation will help to relax your trunk muscles and build strength. It looks as though your arms are like the sails of an old-fashioned wooden windmill, first turning clockwise and then anti-clockwise in the wind.

1. Opening position: Stand with feet shoulder-width apart. Feet parallel and facing 12 o'clock. Chin tucked in slightly. Eyes forwards and relaxed. Shoulders relaxed. Arms hanging loosely down. Fingers gently apart and slightly curved. Palms towards body. Tailbone tucked in. Knees relaxed and slightly bent. Circle arms to head. Turn palms face out to front. Breathe in. Raise arms above head shoulder-width apart. Elbows slightly bent. Clockwise arc arms: Breathe out. Arc arms down in clockwise direction until arms are straight down. Arms shoulder-width apart. Keep elbows rounded. Sink body as arms reach your waist. Follow movement of hands with eyes. Clockwise raise arms.

Turning like a windmill

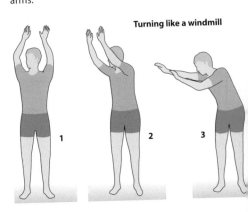

1   2   3

2. Breathe in. Bring arms up in clockwise direction until arms are straight up. Arms shoulder-width apart. Keep elbows rounded.

3. Raise body as the arms reach the waist. Follow movement of hands with eyes and head. Repeat: clockwise lower arms through clockwise raised arms four to six times. Change direction of turn: Breathe out. Bring arms down in clockwise direction until arms are straight down. Arms shoulder-width apart. Keep elbows rounded. Sink body as the arms reach your waist. Follow movement of hands with eyes. Now do the same moves, except in an anti-clockwise direction. Repeat: anti-clockwise lower arms through anti-clockwise raised arms four to six times. Return to starting position: Breathe in. Raise and straighten the body. Let arms return to sides. Palms facing legs.

Exercise 3. Turning the waist
(also known as Beautiful woman turns the waist)
This exercise loosens the back for other exercises, and helps with tight muscles in general. It also helps to strengthen the back. Remember to keep your rotational circles small.

1. Opening position: same as for Turning like a windmill in a calm breeze. Cover kidneys: Place palms on back so that the heel of the palm is roughly at waist height over the kidneys.

2. Straighten knees but avoid locking them. Clockwise hip rotation: Push left hip out to left, bend upper torso slightly right.

3. Push hips forwards and allow upper body to bend backwards slightly.

4. Push right hip out to right and then bend your body slightly to the left. Push bottom backwards and allow body to bend forwards slightly. Repeat: clockwise hip rotation six times. Anti-clockwise hip rotation: Push right hip out to right and bend body slightly left. Push hips forwards and allow upper body to bend backwards slightly.

5. Push left hip out to left, bend upper torso slightly right. Push bottom backwards and allow body to bend forward slightly. Repeat: anti-clockwise hip rotation six times. Return to starting position: Breathe in. Raise and straighten body.

6. Bring arms to hang loosely at sides. Palms should face thighs.

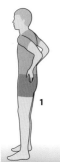

1

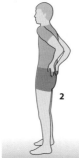

2

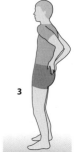

3

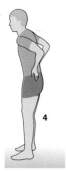

4

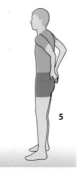

5

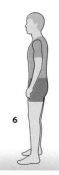

6

Turning the waist

BACK RELIEF THROUGH ACUPUNCTURE

Acupuncture, a branch of Traditional Chinese Medicine (TCM) uses thin, hollow needles to regulate the flow of vital energy, known as *qi* (*see* p. 172). Stimulating acupuncture points is thought to release blockages in this energy flow which cause pain. Needles will be inserted at different points on your body, often on the wrists, ankles and feet, back and abdomen. You shouldn't feel anything apart from a mild tingling sensation or slight soreness. A number of needles may be used, and occasionally moxibustion takes place (burning herbs) at the site. Finger pressure may be used on acupuncture points (acupressure) instead, or 'cupping' is used, where suction cups are placed on the skin to increase circulation. You may get benefits after just one treatment, but often a course of six to ten treatments is likely, especially for chronic problems. Two studies published in the *British Medical Journal* in 2006 found acupuncture to be both cost – and clinically effective in the treatment of back pain.

Self-help

Acupuncture must be undertaken by a registered, experienced practitioner, but you can stimulate a few key points yourself using finger pressure. Press firmly and deeply for 30–60 seconds.

BACK RELIEF THROUGH REFLEXOLOGY

Reflexology is related to acupuncture and acupressure, and involves applying pressure to points on the feet and hands, to stimulate the body's own healing system. Reflexologists believe that parts of the body are reflected on the feet and hands, and that applying pressure to these points can improve physical and emotional health.

Depending on the points chosen, therapists can use the therapy to ease tension, reduce inflammation, improve circulation and eliminate toxins. Smaller studies have found that reflexology is effective, over a course of treatments, for back strains, sciatica and headaches.

Feet as mirrors of the body

According to reflexology, each foot represents half of the body, the left and right foot corresponding to the left and right side of the body. The following divisions of the feet refer to these corresponding parts of the body:

Toes: head and neck
Balls of the feet: chest, lungs, shoulders
Arch (upper part): diaphragm to waist area
Arch (lower part): waist to pelvic area
Heel: pelvic area/sciatic nerve

Inner foot: spine
Outer foot: arm, shoulders, hips, legs, knees, lower back
Ankle area: pelvic area, reproductive organs

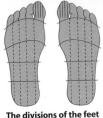

The divisions of the feet and the areas of the body to which they refer (*see* p.179–80).

There are a variety of different techniques used to 'work' the reflex areas of the feet to release blockages and stimulate healing. Usually the thumb and occasionally the index finger are used in small, controlled movements, using different pressure. The emphasis is on being 'firm' but not hard or painful.

Thumbwalking is done with the pad of the thumb. Bend your thumb and rest your other fingers around the foot on which you are working. Press your thumb into the reflex point you want to treat, then release some of the pressure. Slide your thumb along like a caterpillar, stop and press again. Press on the precise area, keeping your movements slow and rhythmic.

Fingerwalking is similar, but is done with the side of the index finger, using your thumb and other three fingers for support.

Rotating involves pressing your thumb into the reflex point while you support the foot with your other hand. Press and rotate your thumb into the reflex point, using your other fingers for support on the other side of the foot.

Flexing involves holding the toes with one hand while you press into the desired point with your other thumb. Gently bend the foot backwards and forwards, so that your thumb presses and releases the point in a rhythmic fashion.

Self-help

It's worth seeing a reflexologist, who can fine-tune treatment and even make a diagnosis through your feet. There are, however, some quick and easy ways to use the reflex points at home. It's worth investing in a good book on reflexology, or downloading a full map of the feet (see **www.aboutreflexology.com**), to ensure that you are hitting the right reflex points.

Your spine

Tilt your foot slightly outwards. Thumbwalk the length of the reflex area for the spine (inner foot) from the base of the heel up to the area at the base of the toenail. This is the point for the first cervical (neck) vertebra.

Switch your hand position. Thumb- or fingerwalk the area at the base of your big toe from several directions.

Switch hands and thumbwalk down the entire spinal reflex area (inner foot), using the top of the other hand for support.

Thumbwalk horizontally across the edge of the foot, starting at the base of the heel and moving upwards.

Stop, rotate and pivot every few millimetres, which will help to ensure that you get every point that corresponds to the 26 vertebrae in the spine.

Sciatica

Thumbwalk across the sciatic nerve line on the bottom of the heel (which sits about 2 cm/1 in or so up from the back of the heel, on the sole of your foot, and runs horizontally across the foot). Fingerwalk up the outside of your foot, along the Achilles tendon (which runs up the back of your ankle). Reverse hands for working on the other foot.

Alternatively, press points that feel a bit tender on your feet along the spine area (tenderness on the feet is often an indication that there is a problem with the corresponding part of the body). Hold with your thumb for five minutes, and repeat as required.

BACK RELIEF THROUGH HYDROTHERAPY

Hydrotherapy is the use of water (including steam and ice) for therapeutic purposes. A sauna, the use of hot or cold compresses, soaking in a bathtub or spa and applying ice to an injury are all forms of hydrotherapy.

Hydrotherapy relieves back pain by loosening the muscles and ridding the body of toxins that produce pain and inflammation. Studies have shown that people who soak in a hot tub or warm bath have less stiffness, more flexibility, and tend to use less pain medication.

Generally, heat quiets and soothes the body, slowing down the activity of internal organs. Cold, in contrast, stimulates and invigorates, increasing internal activity. If you are experiencing tense muscles and anxiety, a hot shower or bath is in order. If you are feeling tired and stressed, you might want to try taking a warm shower or bath followed by a short, invigorating cold shower to help stimulate your body and mind.

When you submerge yourself in a bath, pool or whirlpool, you experience a kind of weightlessness. Your body is relieved from the constant pull of gravity. Water also has a hydrostatic effect. It has a massage-like feeling as the water gently kneads your body. Water, in motion, stimulates touch receptors on the skin, boosting blood circulation and releasing tight muscles.

Most spas, gyms and even salons now offer hydrotherapy treatments, as do many physio-therapists; alternatively, you can take matters into your own hands and undertake your own treatment at home.

> Do not use any hot water treatments on new injuries; ice should be used for the first 24–48 hours to relieve inflammation and swelling (*see* p. 93).

Douching: To douche your back, use a hose hooked up to your bathtub tap. Direct the stream of warm water over the painful area and towards the heart. The water should not splash, but rather wash gently over the skin. Hold for as long as is comfortable.

Saunas and steam baths help relieve mild back pain by stimulating the flow of blood, which relieves the pain of strained or injured muscles. Avoid using a sauna if you suffer from diabetes or are pregnant, and do not stay in longer than 15 minutes. Drink plenty of water to prevent dehydration, which is one cause of back pain.

Warm baths are excellent for relieving back pain. Fill the tub with about 15 cm (6 in) of tepid water and get in. Gradually add hot water until the water level in the tub reaches your naval, and relax into the water with a support for your head (a rolled-up towel will do). The water should be hot enough to feel comfortable, but not cause the skin to redden. Aromatherapy oils can enhance the effect (*see* pp. 156–7), but only use 1–2 drops.

Heat wraps can be useful to loosen areas of localised tension and reduce pain. Moisten a cloth with warm water, wring it out, and wrap it snugly around the painful area of your back. Then wrap up, first in a dry cloth and then, over this, in a blanket. Relax. Aromatherapy oils can be added to the water (about five drops) for maximum effect.

Bathing in a warm bath for just five minutes in the morning will help to loosen muscles and stiffness from sleep; in the evening, the same routine (warm, not hot water, which can be too stimulating and prevent healthy sleep) can relax muscles that have been tensed during the day, and help to soothe pain.

FURTHER RESOURCES

General

BackCare: The Charity for Healthier Backs
16 Elmtree Road, Teddington, Middlesex TW11 8ST
020 8977 5474 Helpline: 0845 130 2704
(local rate)
www.backpain.org

Action on Pain
01760 725993 Painline: 0845 603 1593
www.action-on-pain.co.uk

Support and advice for those affected by pain

The British Pain Society
020 7631 8870 info@britishpainsociety.org
www.britishpainsociety.org
Representative body for healthcare professionals
and scientists involved in the management and
understanding of pain

NHS Direct
0845 4647 (24 hours)
www.nhsdirect.nhs.uk
Good, general information, plus help with
diagnosis and understanding treatment

Brain and Spine Foundation
Helpline: 0808 808 1000
www.brainandspine.org.uk

A good resource on the web, and their helpline can provide assistance and advice with all spine conditions

British Association for Counselling and Psychotherapy

BACP House, 35–37 Albert Street, Rugby, Warkwickshire CV21 2SG

0870 443 5252 **www.bacp.co.uk**

This organisation produces a directory of qualified counsellors and psychotherapists

Websites

www.spine-health.com

Excellent site with a huge range of information on all types of pain treatments, both conventional and complementary

www.back.com

A good American site with information, advice, links and patient stories

www.spineuniverse.com

This site hosts more than 5,000 pages on every conceivable aspect of back pain. Well worth a visit

www.bbc.co.uk/health/conditions/back_pain

A good basic introduction to back pain, with some useful links and tips

www.babycentre.co.uk

Excellent resource for back pain in pregnancy

Therapies

Chartered Society of Physiotherapy
14 Bedford Row, London WC1R 4ED
020 7306 6218 **www.csp.org.uk**

The Organisation of Chartered Physiotherapists in Private Practice
Cedar House, The Bell Plantation, Watling Street, Towcester, Northants NN12 6GX
01327 354441 **www.physiofirst.org.uk**

General Council for Massage Therapy
27 Old Gloucester Street, London WC1N 3XX
0870 850 4452 **www.gcmt.org.uk**

Qi gong Southwest
www.qigong-southwest.co.uk

Pilates Foundation UK
PO Box 57060, London EC4P 4XB
07071 781 859 **www.pilatesfoundation.com**

General Osteopathic Council
176 Tower Bridge Road, London SE1 3LU
020 7357 6655 **www.osteopathy.org.uk**

British Chiropractic Association
59 Castle Street, Reading, Berkshire RG1 7SN
0118 950 5950 **www.chiropractic-uk.co.uk**

General Chiropractic Council
44 Wicklow Street, London WC1X 9HL
020 7713 5155 **www.gcc-uk.org**

The Scottish Chiropractic Association
Laigh Hatton Farm, Old Greenock Road, Bishopton,

Renfrewshire PA7 5PB
01505 863151 **www.sca-chiropractic.org**

British Acupuncture Council
63 Jeddo Road, London W12 9HQ
020 8735 0400 **www.acupuncture.org.uk**

British Medical Acupuncture Society
BMAS House, 3 Winnington Court, Northwich,
Cheshire CW8 1AQ
01606 786782 **www.medical-acupuncture.co.uk**

**The British Complementary Medicine Association
(BCMA)**
P.O. Box 5122, Bournemouth BH8 0WG
0845 345 5977 **www.bcma.co.uk**

Association of Reflexologists
5 Fore Street, Taunton, Somerset TA1 1HX
0870 5673320 **www.aor.org.uk**

The British Wheel of Yoga
BWY Central Office, 25 Jermyn Street, Sleaford,
Lincolnshire NG34 7RU
01529 306851 **www.bwy.org.uk**

The Hypnotherapy Association
14 Crown Street, Chorley, Lancashire PR7 1DX
01257 262124
www.thehypnotherapyassociation. co.uk

The Society of Teachers of the Alexander Technique
1st Floor, Linton House, 39–51 Highgate Road,
London NW5 1RS
0845 230 7828 **www.stat.org.uk**

INDEX

page numbers in **bold**
refer to illustrations

abdominal exercises 74
  98, 113
absenteeism 4
acupressure 178
acupuncture 26, 85-6, 178
adrenaline 39, 42
aerobic exercises, low-
  impact 25, 29, 42, 130
affirmations, positive
  159-61
aging 9-10, 29, 33-4, 63
Alexander Technique
  47-59, 131-2
  classes 53
  positions 47, 49-50,
    53-9, **54**, **56**, **58**
  primary control 47, 49
  and self-awareness 50-2
ALTENS 85-6
alternate nostril
  breathing 123
alternative therapies
  140-85
  consultations 142-3
  examinations 143
  finding a practitioner
    141-2
  treatments 144-85
anatomy 7-8
anti-convulsants 24
anti-inflammatories 23-
  5, 63, 92-3, 157, 184
antibiotics 24
antidepressants, tricyclic
  24
antioxidants 6, 33, 61, 63
arm swings 173
arrow 115
aspirin 23

asthma 23
autogenic relaxation
  167-8

babies 38, 78-80
baby carriers 80
'back against the wall'
  58-9, **58**
back extensions 119
back extensors 115
bags 31
ballerina arms (exercise)
  116, **116**
baths 90-1, 184-5
beds 64-7, 68-70, **68**
bending 51
beta carotene 62
body scanning 171
bone scans 20-1
braces 26
brain 6
breastfeeding 23, 80
breathing 108, 110, 121-3,
  170-1
bridging 113
British Medical Journal 178
bromelain 62
buoyancy 138

calcium 15, 33, 60
car seats, heated 92
cat (exercise) 117, 124
cauda equina 16
causes of back pain 10-16
cerebrospinal fluid 6
chair raises 97-8
Chinese medicine 143,
  172, 178
chiropractic 26, 144-5
chronic pain 168
cobra (exercise) 124-5,
  125
codeine 24
cognitive behaviour

therapy (CBT) 163-4
cognitive restructuring
  162-3
cold treatments 92-3,
  157, 183, 184
collagen 61
complete breath
  (exercise) 123
computerized
  tomography (CT) 19
core muscles 55-7, 76, 82,
  110-12
counter-irritants 23
cupping (acupuncture) 1
cupping (massage) 153
cycle of pain 40, 41-2

degenerative condition:
  14, 15
degenerative processes
  9-10, 33-4, 63
dehydration 34, 96
diagnosis 6, 17-21
diet 142
discogenic back pain 1
discography 19
discs 7-8, 14, 16, 88
  artificial 27
decompression 27
degeneration 33, 34
  physical exercise for
    53-4, 136
  prolapsed (herniated)
    12-13, **12**, 34, 40
  and sedentary
    lifestyles 31
  and sleep 66, 67
  tests for 17-18
distraction 161-2
doctors 10-11, 17-20, 8
douching 184
draining 151, **151**
driving posture 34-6
electrical stimulation a

electrodiagnostic
  procedures 20
electromyography (EMG) 20
emotions, and pain 40-1
endorphins 42, 86, 87-8, 95
epidurals 25
essential fatty acids
  (EFAs) 62-3
essential oils 149-50,
  156-7, 185
ETPS 85, **85**
everyday back relief 38-80
evoked potential
  studies 20

facet joints 7, 9, 25
fibromyalgia 15-16
'fight or flight' mode 39, 165
forward bends 129, **129**
fracture 15
friction strokes 152

gate theory 83
gliding 150-1
GPR 88
GS 84-5

hacking 152-3
hamstring stretch 119
'hand and knees' 76
head position 47, 49-50
Health and Safety
  Executive 4
heat treatments 25, 89-93,
  183, 185
heel raises 106, **106**
hip exercises 101-2, **101**, 119
hormones 39, 72, 165
hot water bottles 90
humping and hollowing 74
hydrostatic pressure
  138, 183-4
hydrotherapy 183-5
hypnosis 168-9
ibuprofen 23, 63

ice massage 93, 157
ice packs 25, 93, 184
IFC 84
imagery 162
inflammation 14, 22
  see also
    anti-inflammatories
injury 9, 15

jogging, water 139

kneading 151
knee to chest (exercise)
  98, 126, 139

labour 57, 72, 75-8
leg crossing 50-1
leg exercises 29, 97, **97**, 139
lifting 32, 37, 78-80
ligaments 72-3, 78
lumbar stabilisation 104

McKenzie exercises 99
McKenzie extension 100-1
magnesium 62
manganese 61
manipulation 26, 144-5
mantras 171
massage 43, 73, 145, 148-57
  routine 153-5, **154**
  techniques 150-3, **151**
mattresses 64-6
medical help 22-5, 81-93
meditation 170-1, 172-3
meridians 172
mind-body relationship 158
missionary position 70-1
mobilisation 145
monkey position 55-7,
  56, 77
morning stiffness 64, 68-9,
  185
MRI 19-20
muscle relaxants 23
muscles

elasticity 91-2
stiffness 11, 15, 64,
  68-9, 185
strains and sprains 11
tension 39-40, 146, 149
musculo-skeletal
  system 144
music 43
myelograms 19

naproxen 23
neck stretches 118
nerve-conduction
  studies 20
nerves 8, 13
nervous system 8, 165
neutral spine posture 111
NICE 81
NSAIDs 23
numbness 13
nutrition 33, 60-3

opiates 24
osteoarthritis 14, 136
osteomyelitis 15
osteopathy 26, 144, 146-7
osteoporosis 15, 33, 60,
  130, 147
over-the-counter drugs
  22-3

Paget's disease 14, 16
pain perception 39, 158, 165
pain relief 81-93
pain-spasm cycle 23
palm tree 127-8, **128**
paracetamol 23
paresthesia 83
passive therapies 25
pedometers 130
pelvic floor exercises
  74-5, 76
pelvic girdle pain 73
pelvic tilting 75-6
percussive strokes 152-3

phosphorous 33, 60
physical exercise 25,
    28-9, 42, 79, 94-139
    advantages of 95
    types of 96-139
physical therapy 25, 26
physiotherapy 87-8
Pilates 76, 107-18, **112**,
    114, **116**
pillows 64, 66-7
pinching/plucking 153
Piriformis stretch 102, **102**
plough 125-6, **126**
positive thinking 32, 159-61
posture 8, 29-37, 44-59,
    45, 111, 131-2, **131**
pregnancy 23, 38, 72-6,
    117, 150
prevalence 4
prevention 6, 28-37, 38-80
previous problems 39-40
progressive muscle
    relaxation 166-7
pronation 134
prostaglandins 63
Psoas major stretch 102-3
psychological
    treatments 158-64
psychosomatic illness 40-1
pulling technique **151**, 152

Qi Gong 171, 172-7, **174**,
    177

referred pain 9
reflexes 17, 149
reflexology 179-82, **180**
relaxation 43, 121, 164-9
remedial massage 148
rheumatoid arthritis 14, 147
rhythmic activity 162
rollups 113-15, **114**

sacroiliac joint blocks 25
sacroiliitis 16

saunas 90, 184
saw exercise 117-18
sciatica 13, 18, 40, 73, 182
scissor spreads 139
sedentary lifestyles 48-9
self-awareness 50-2
self-help 90-2, 178, 181-2
sex 64, 70-1
shoes 31, 50, 132-3
sitting 30-1, 48-52
sleep 32, 43, 64-7
smoking 33
SNRBs 25
spinal cord 6-7
spinal injections 24-5
spinal stenosis 13-14, 66
spinal twist 127, **127**
spine 49, 182-3
    anatomy 6-7, **9**
    problems 9-11, 34
    widening and
    lengthening 53-4, **54**
spondylolisthesis 14-15
spooning 71
sprains 11
spurs (new bone) 14
steam baths 184
steroids 24-5
stiffness 11, 14, 15, 64,
    68-9, 185
straight leg test 17-18
strain 11, 98
strengthening exercises
    25, 29, 97-102
stress 29, 38-43, 142, 165
stretching 25, 29, 42-3,
    79, 107-19, 138
support belts 74
surgery 27
swimming 136-9
Swiss balls 87-8, 102-5,
    105-6
symphysis pubis 73

TENS 25, 26, 83-4

tests 17-20
thermography 21
thumbwalking 180, 181-2
topical analgesics 23
transverse abdominus 113
travelling posture 37
trigger points 145, 155
turning like a windmill...
    173-5, **174**
turning the waist 175-6, **17**

ultrasound 21, 25
urinary problems 16

vertebrae 7, 9, 27
visualisation, creative 166
vital energy (qi) 172-3, 178
vitality breath 122
vitamins 33, 60, 61-2

walking 46, 130-6, **131**, 13
wall slides 97
wall squats 106, **106**
warm-ups 28, 91
warning signs 33-4
water beds 66
water exercise 136-9
water intake 34, 96
wear and tear 12, 63
weight 33, 72
weight-bearing exercise 7
work 4, 29-31
work surfaces 29, 30-1
wringing technique **15**,
    152

x-rays 18-19, 144

yoga 120-9, 171
    breathing 121-3
    positions 124-9

zip and hollow exercise
    112, **112**